Pelvic Floor Dysfunction - Symptoms, Causes, and Treatment

Edited by Ran Pang

Published in London, United Kingdom

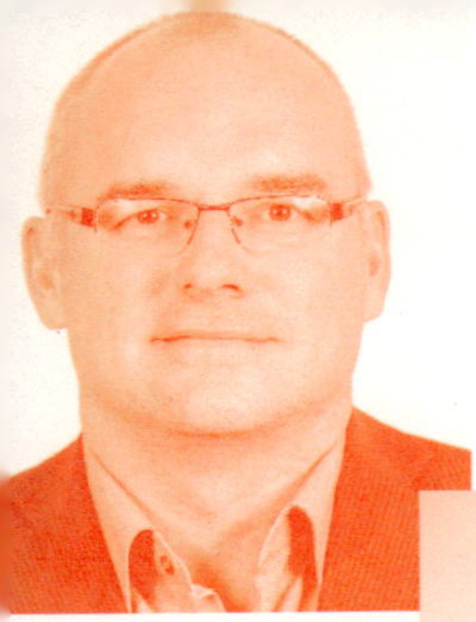
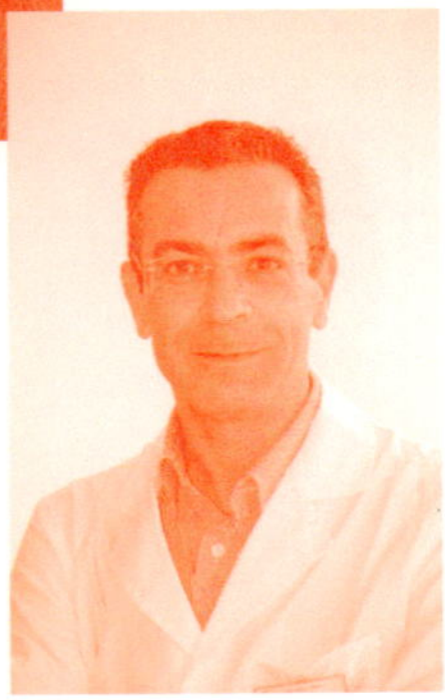
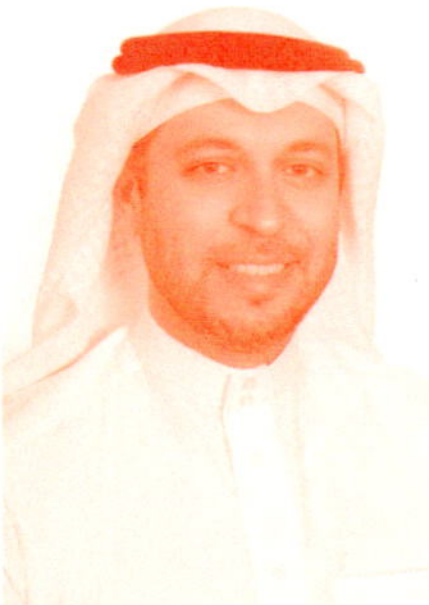
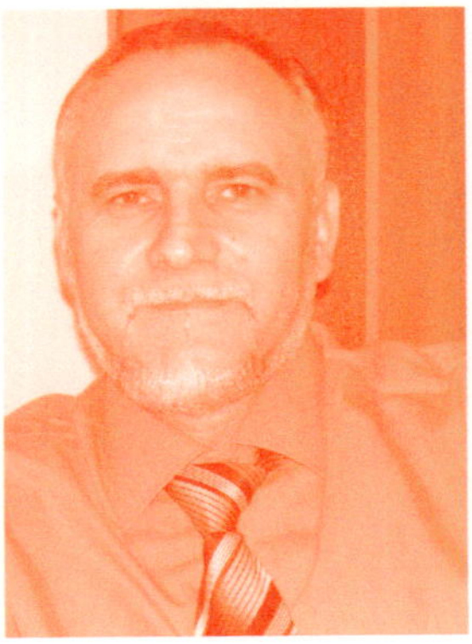
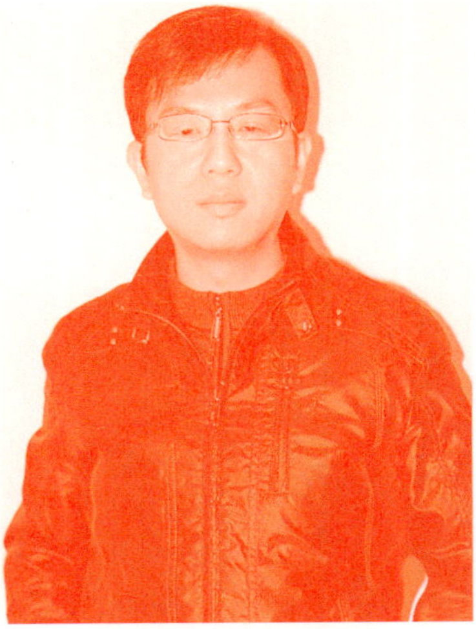
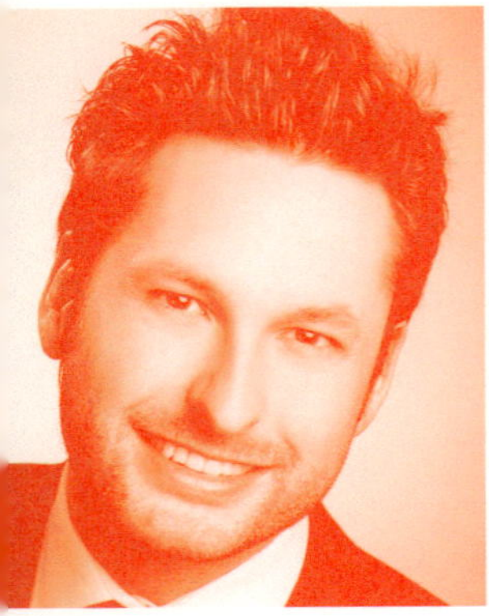
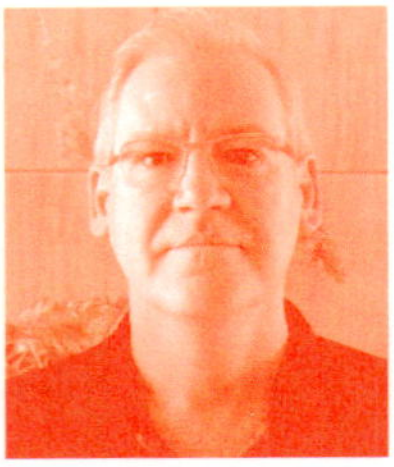

IntechOpen

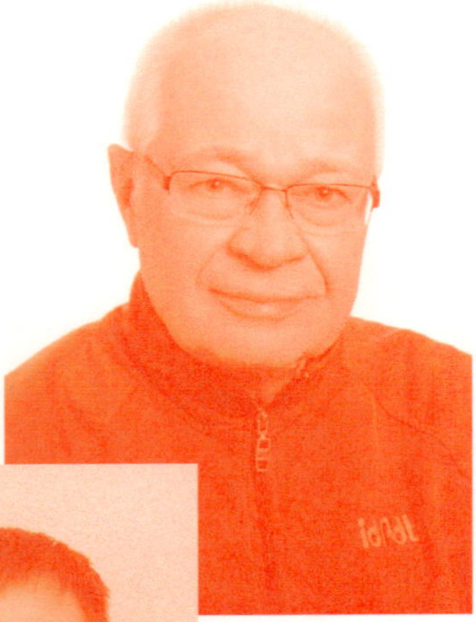
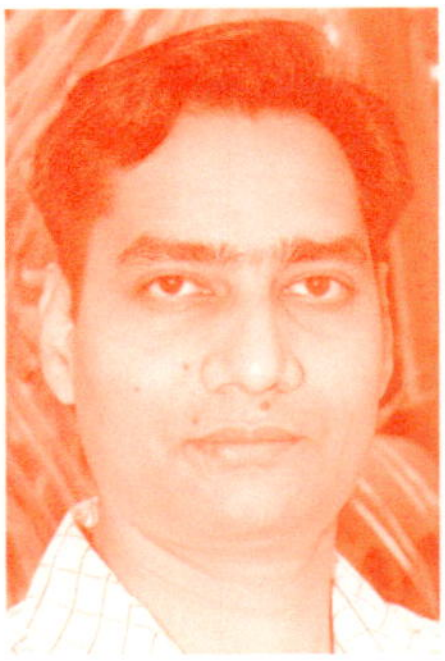
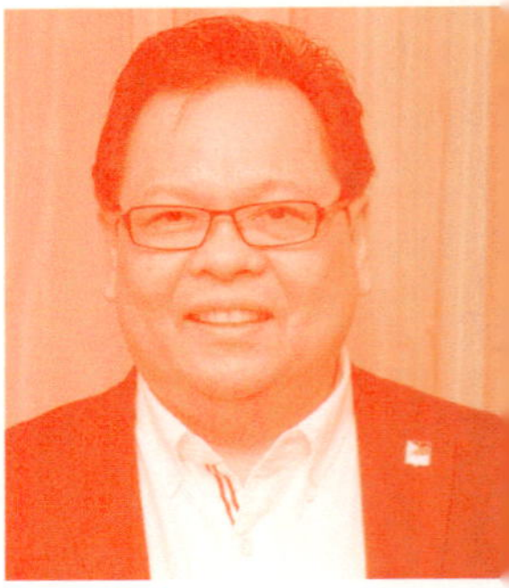
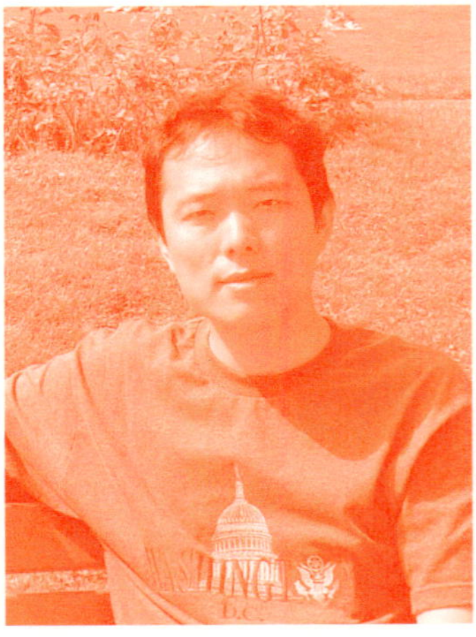
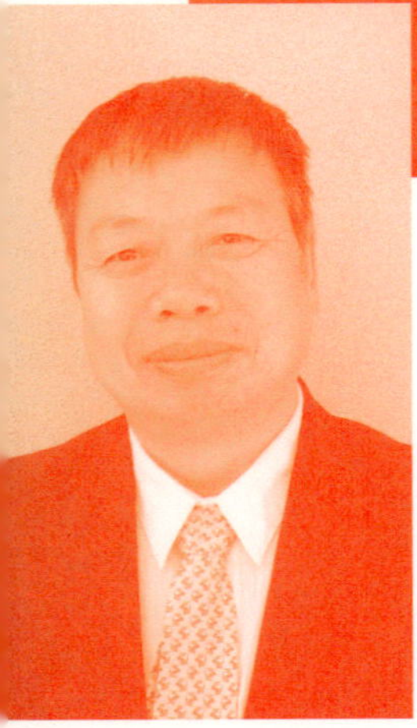
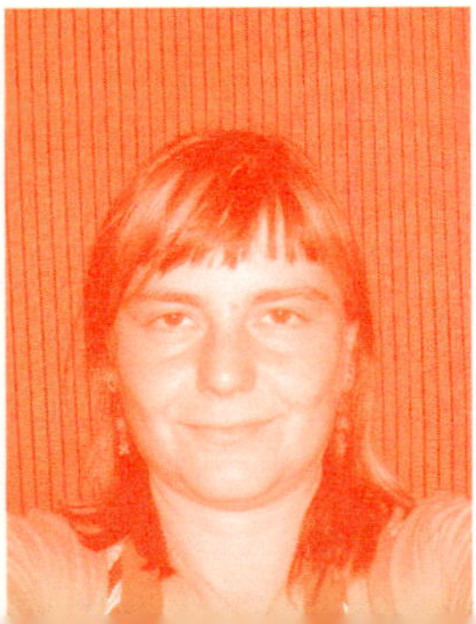

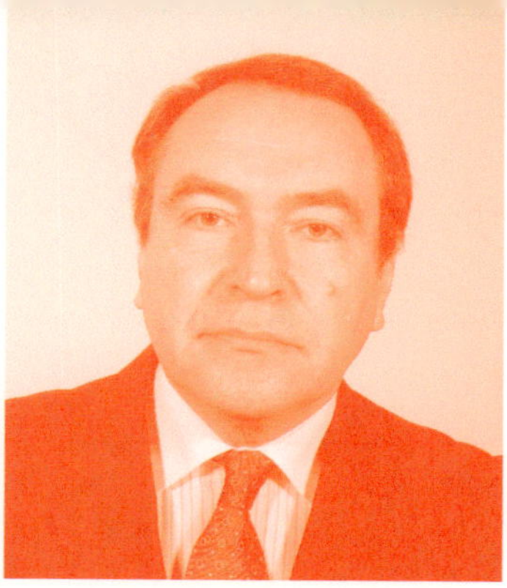
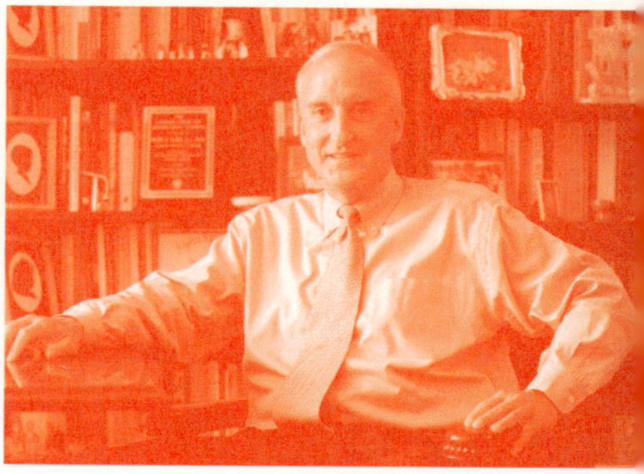
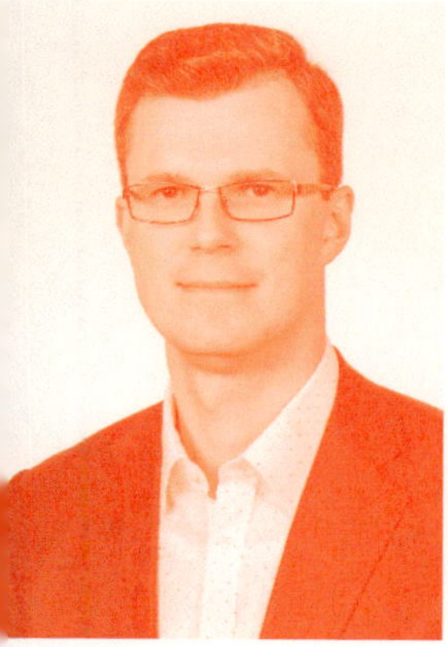
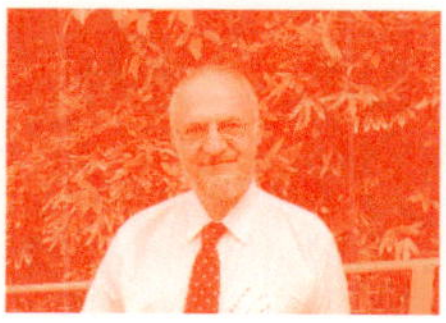
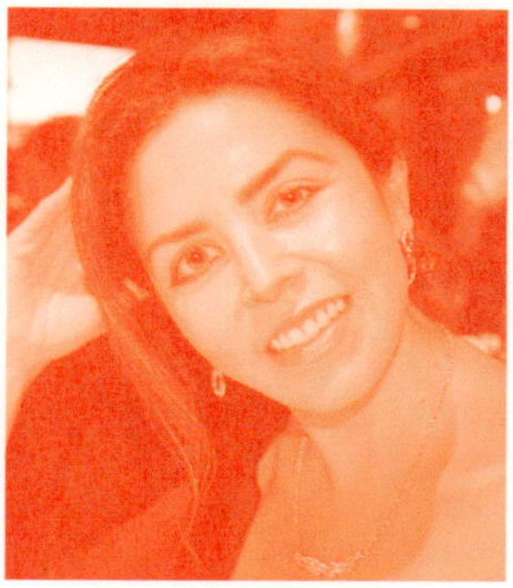

Supporting open minds since 2005

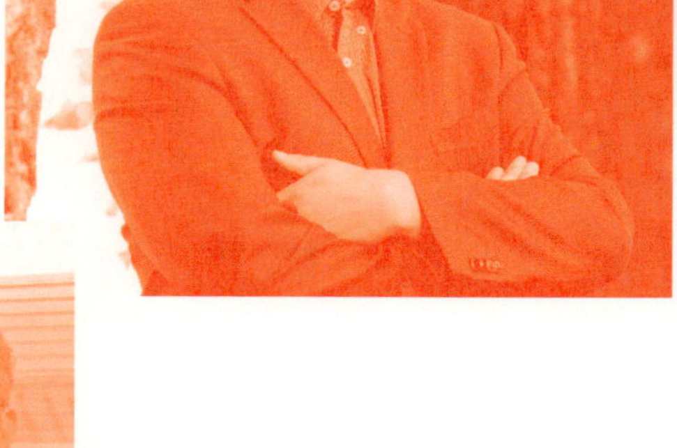
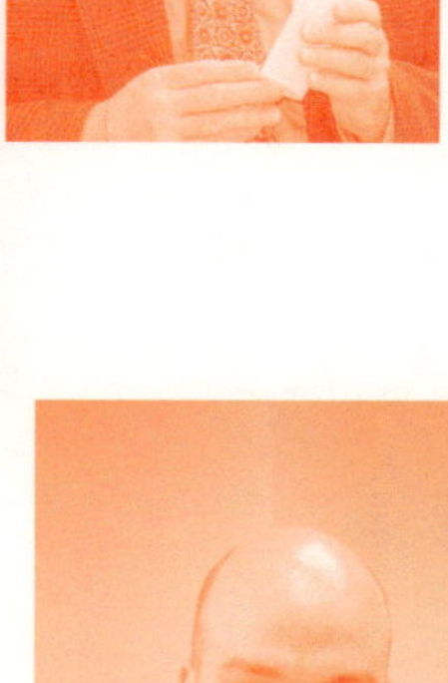
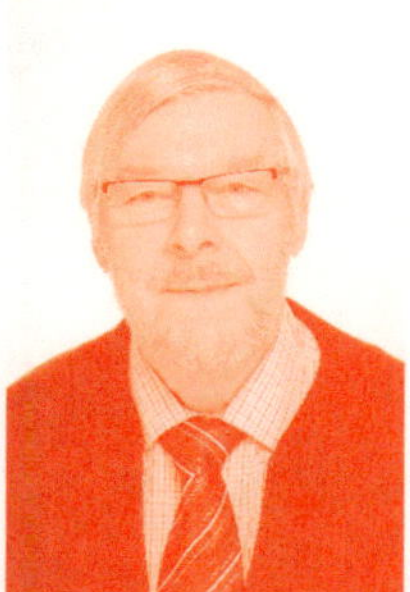
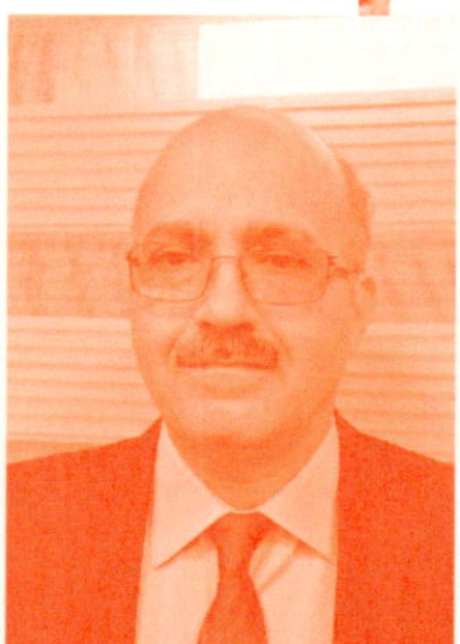
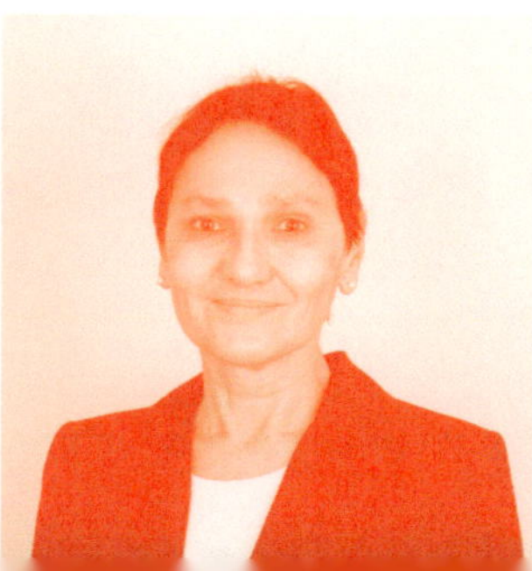
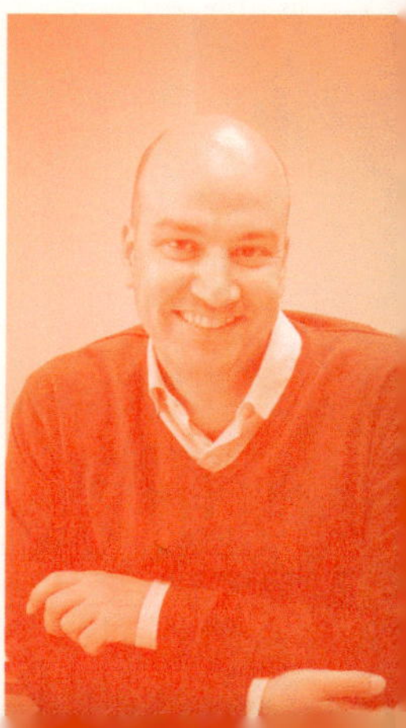

Pelvic Floor Dysfunction - Symptoms, Causes, and Treatment
http://dx.doi.org/10.5772/intechopen.94692
Edited by Ran Pang

Contributors
Monika Sorfova, Eva Tlapakova, Cristhel K. K. Fagerstrom-Sade, Marcela M. Gurovich, Sara Parada-Ibañez, Pablo Ortega-Plancic, Jaime Roa-Burgos, Fabian Vasquez-Vergara, Esther Ayala-Pérez, Jorge Rodriguez-Suazo, Rodrigo Garcia-Baquero, Cristina Margarita Fernández-Ávila, Ana Victoria Ojeda Claro, Blanca Madurga Patuel, Jose Luis Alvarez-Ossorio, Heltty Heltty, Ratna Sitorus, Nury Nusdwinuringtyas, Evi Martha, Vesna D. Zivkovic, Ivona Stankovic, Dragan Zlatanovic, Lidija Dimitrijevic, Hristina Colovic, Natasa Savic, Shigeo Horie, Takuro Kobayashi, Toshiyuki China, Naoko Takasawa, Fumitaka Shimizu, Julius Fink, Tomohiro Imai, Kyu-Sung Lee, Kwang Jin Ko, Isabell Link, Christian Fünfgeld

First published in London, United Kingdom, 2022 by IntechOpen
IntechOpen is the global imprint of INTECHOPEN LIMITED, registered in England and Wales, registration number: 11086078, 5 Princes Gate Court, London, SW7 2QJ, United Kingdom
Printed in Croatia

British Library Cataloguing-in-Publication Data
A catalogue record for this book is available from the British Library

Additional hard and PDF copies can be obtained from orders@intechopen.com

Pelvic Floor Dysfunction - Symptoms, Causes, and Treatment
Edited by Ran Pang
p. cm.
Print ISBN 978-1-83969-361-8
Online ISBN 978-1-83969-362-5
eBook (PDF) ISBN 978-1-83969-363-2

For EU product safety concerns:
IN TECH d.o.o., Prolaz Marije Krucifikse Kozulić 3, 51000 Rijeka, Croatia, info@intechopen.com or visit our website at intechopen.com.

Meet the editor

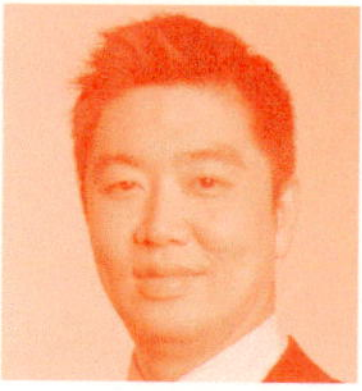

Ran Pang is a consultant urologist and leader in functional urology and urodynamics at Guang'anmen hospital, China Academy of Chinese Medical Sciences. After completing residency training, he was accepted to a clinical fellowship with Peking University in 2005. Subsequently, he joined a research fellowship at Mayo Clinic, USA, in 2011, and a urodynamic fellowship at Dalhousie University, Canada, in 2015. As a leading expert, prof. Pang also serves on several international organizations as well as local professional committees, such as chair of the Publication and Communication Committee, International Continence Society, and vice-chair of the Pelvic Floor Disorder Group of Urology Committee, Chinese Association of Integrative Medicine. Additionally, he received the Albert Nelson Lifetime Achievement award in 2017.

Contents

Preface

Pelvic floor disorders (PFDs) refer to a group of conditions, such as urinary incontinence, fecal incontinence, and pelvic organ prolapse (POP), due to weakened or injured pelvic muscles and connective tissues. The pelvic muscles and connective tissues play an important role in supporting the pelvic organs, including the bowel, bladder, rectum, and in women, the uterus, since they form an anatomical hammock across the floor of the pelvis. Once these muscles or connective tissues are weakened or injured, the function of pelvic organs will be affected and consequently PFDs will occur.

In general, the diagnosis and management of PFDs remain a challenge because the symptoms of PFDs are various. In their chapter, Dr. Isabell Link and Christian Fünfgeld provide us with an outline of female PFDs. They describe not only are the key points of diagnosis, but also therapeutic and preventive strategies.

Understanding pelvic floor muscle activity is the basis for management of PFDs. Several studies focusing on pelvic floor muscle activity have been performed since Dr. Kegel developed an intravaginal device to measure pelvic floor muscle strength in 1948. However, the effect of different positions and breath status on pelvic floor muscle activity is still unclear. In their chapter, Prof. Monika Sorfova and Eva Tlapakova demonstrate the results of their research, which may help clinicians to develop a more efficient protocol of pelvic floor muscle training.

Pregnancy and childbirth are important acquired risk factors for female PFDs. On one hand, pregnancy and childbirth can put excessive strain on the pelvic floor, which may result in pelvic floor muscle fatigue. On the other hand, episiotomy during delivery can directly injury the pelvic muscles and connective tissues. It may minimize the occurrence of PFDs to understand the indication of episiotomy and perform this surgery properly. To understand the knowledge of gynecologists and midwives, Dr. Cristhel K. Fagerstrom-Sade et al. conducted a cross-sectional study in Chile. The results of the study provide valuable evidence in this field.

The management of PFDs mainly depends on the patients' clinical presentation. Basically, conservative therapy is considered the first-line treatment for PFDs. Magnetic stimulation, as a non-invasive therapy, has been one of the most common therapies for treating PFDs. In their chapter, Dr. Shigeo Horie et al. present current evidence in the therapeutic effect of magnetic stimulation on various PFDs. More importantly, they discuss the application of magnetic stimulation in Japan.

Interstitial cystitis/bladder pain syndrome (IC/BPS) is believed to be a kind of complicated PFD. However, because its etiology remains unclear, the diagnostic criteria are confusing, and no definitive treatments are available. Generally, IC/BPS can be classified into two types: Hunner lesion IC/BPS and non-Hunner lesion IC/BPS. It is reported that patients with Hunner lesion IC/BPS have more severe symptoms and lower bladder capacity compared to those with non-Hunner lesion IC/BPS. Thus, management of Hunner lesion IC/BPS seems to be more difficult. In their chapter,

Dr. Kwang Jin Ko and Kyu-Sung Lee not only list currently available treatments but also present evidence for the efficacy of each treatment, which can help clinicians to choose the proper therapeutic strategy.

Post-stroke urinary incontinence is a common PFD in the elderly. It is normally managed as a chronic illness because it is a sequela of stroke. In their chapter, Prof. Heltty Heltty et al. develop an integrated management model that includes a holistic rehabilitation program and continuous care at the patient's home. This therapeutic model may boost patient confidence in overcoming the disease.

Dysfunctional voiding is a common disorder in children. Traditionally, its etiology is attributed to habitual disorder and psychosocial problems. Recently, more and more studies show several factors, including learned behavior, the perpetuation of infantile patterns, maturational delay, and genetic or congenital factors, may contribute to the occurrence of dysfunctional voiding. Despite the development in understanding its etiology, there is no universal treatment so far. In their chapter, Dr. Vesna D. Zivkovic et al. present different rehabilitation protocols in details, which may allow patients to choose multimodal and individualized therapy.

POP is the dropping of the pelvic organs caused by the weakened support of pelvic muscles and connective tissues. Surgery has been the mainstream treatment for POP. In their chapter, Dr. Rodrigo García-Baquero et al. share their experience in managing POP using single-incision mesh and discuss other surgical procedures. Their case study provides important evidence in the safety of the procedure.

In this book, experts and researchers from different countries present the latest evidence in the diagnosis and treatment of PFDs. Although these chapters cannot cover all the aspects of PFDs, they provide readers with important updates. I believe a bright future in this field awaits us.

Ran Pang
Department of Urology,
Guang'anmen Hospital,
China Academy of Chinese Medical Sciences,
Beijing, China

Section 1

Basic Considerations in Pelvic Floor Disorders

Chapter 1

Pelvic Floor Disorders in Females: An Overview on Diagnostics and Therapy

Isabell Link and Christian Fünfgeld

Abstract

Pelvic floor disorders have multifactorial reasons and can have a huge impact on a woman's life. They can result in descensus of bladder, uterus, vagina or rectum and are often accompanied by incontinence. Symptoms like downward pressure, pain, incontinence or bladder voiding dysfunction develop slowly and are still highly taboo. Gynecology differentiates between descensus of the anterior, central and posterior compartment. A descensus in the anterior compartment causes a cystocele, with can either present as a pulsation cystocele or a traction cystocele. A descensus of the apical compartment leads to a uterine prolapse or vaginal stump descensus, while a descensus of the posterior compartment results in a recto- or enterocele. Urinary incontinence can be divided into stress and urge incontinence. The most important tool for the diagnosis of pelvic floor disorders is the clinical examination. Regarding the therapy of pelvic floor disorders, conservative therapy measures should first be offered. If these fail, an individually optimized surgical therapy should follow. The spectrum of surgical possibilities has expanded considerably in the last three decades. In particular, implanting alloplastic meshes has improved long-term stability. Finally, preventive measures also play a central role.

Keywords: pelvic floor disorders, prolpase, zystocele, rectocele, incontinence, treatment

1. Introduction

The pelvic floor has an important holding and support function in a woman's body. If this substantial holding apparatus suffers from disorders, this can have a huge impact on a woman's quality of live, as taking part in everyday life can be considerably restricted by pelvic floor disorders. The pelvic floor consists of fasciae (endopelvic fascia, rectovaginal septum, perirectal fascia), ligaments (ligg. Sacrouterina, arcus tendineus etc.) and muscles (pelvic diaphragma, urogenital diaphragma), which are already exposed to a high load due to the upright gait. Other events in a woman's life like injuries, chronic overload or giving birth contribute to further stress on the pelvic floor and can lead to disorders. Vaginal delivery, an event most women experience at least once in their lifetime, can lead to damage to connective tissue, ligaments and muscles up to tearing of muscular structures and stretching of pelvic nerves. Hereditary connective tissue weakness contributes further to the weakness of the pelvic floor. In summary, pelvic floor disorders have multifactorial reasons and can result in descensus of the bladder, the uterus, the vagina or the rectum as well as incontinence. In most women, symptoms occur in an advanced stage, with the woman being able to compensate the symptoms through training of the pelvic floor muscles in earlier stages. As muscle strength decreases, the level of suffering increases, while fecal and urinary incontinence may also occur at earlier stages. Women present to their gynecologist with urinary incontinence or prolapse symptoms, while anal incontinence is still highly taboo.

2. Incidence and epidemiology

The incidence of asymptomatic prolapse is high, with approximately 50% of the women after vaginal delivery having an asymptomatic descensus in gynecological examination. 8–30% of the women report symptoms of pelvic floor disorders [1]. The most common symptom of pelvic floor disorders are symptoms related to urination with up to 40% of women suffering from urinary incontinence and bladder voiding dysfunction [2]. The prevalence of pelvic floor disorders rises with age, with 9.7% of the women aged between 20 and 39 years and 49.7% of the women at the age of 80 or older reporting at least one pelvic floor disorders in an US-American study. 12.8% of women who never had given birth reported urinary incontinence, while women after one delivery experienced urinary incontinence in 18.4%. This number increases to 32.4% after three births. The frequency of pelvic floor disorders rises regardless of the mode of delivery, while instrumental delivery bears the highest risk to develop pelvic floor disorder [3]. In general, the incidence of pelvic floor disorders is higher in Eurasian females compared to African females and also higher in overweight women compared to women with normal weight. About every 9th woman will need descensus surgery in her lifetime [4], with 29% needing relapse surgery [5].

3. Etiology and pathogenesis

Pelvic floor disorders are multifactorial. Damage to the muscles, ligaments and fasciae of the pelvic floor leads to loss of function. Human's upright gait already leads to a certain stress on the pelvic floor. Furthermore, chronic overload in the context of prolonged high physical stress, obstetric trauma and hereditary connective tissue weakness can lead to prolapse. While chronic overload usually leads to overstretching of the pelvic floor's muscles and fasciae, birth trauma causes tearing of these structures. While the risk for developing a pelvic floor disorder is highest for instrumental delivery, cesarean section and pregnancy itself already increase the risk. Still, prevalence of prolapse is approximately twice as high in women after vaginal birth compared to women after cesarean section [6]. Stress urinary incontinence usually occurs after the bladder neck loses support and through urethraurethral hypermobility as well as weakness of the urinary sphincter. The pathogenesis of urgency incontinence is more complex, which makes it also more complicated to treat. Mechanism contributing to urgency incontinence are detrusor overactivity, poor detrusor compliance and bladder hypersensitivity [7]. Furthermore, neurological damage of somatic and vegetative nerves should always be considered as a reason for pelvic floor disorders. Pelvic floor prolapse usually only become symptomatic in later stages (when reaching to the vaginal introitus) or when accompanied by anal or urinary incontinence.

4. Definition and classification

Types of Pelvic floor disorders are pelvic floor prolapse and both urinary and fecal incontinence.

4.1 Pelvic floor prolapse

Gynecology differentiates between descensus of the anterior (cystocele), central (uterine prolapse or vaginal stump descensus) and posterior (rectocele, enterocele) compartment, often affecting several compartments at the same time. In addition, a classification according to the level of the defect according to DeLancey takes place:

- Level I—Suspension of the upper third of the vagina, Parakolpium. Damage in this area is referred to as apical or central defects.

- Level II—pubocervical fascia, fixation of the vagina. Damage in this area can lead to paravaginal, lateral defects (cysto- and rectocele).

- Level III—pubourerhral ligaments. Damage in this area leads to stress incontinence [8].

The classification of prolapse is based on the height of the hymenal hem (ICS/IUGA-classification). For example, a rectocele is classified according to the descent of the posterior vaginal wall. If this remains above the hymenal hem during pushing, a stage 1 is present (>1 cm proximal of the hymenal hem). If it descends to the hymenal hem, stage 2 (± 1 cm proximal or distal the hymenal hem), and below that, stage 3(>1 cm distal of the hymenal hem). Stage 4 describes a total prolapse of the uterus and/or the vagina. The same applies to cystocele or descensus uteri [8].

4.1.1 Descensus of the anterior compartment

A descensus in the anterior compartment causes a cystocele. The anterior vaginal wall is connected to the bladder by a layer of connective tissue (fascia endopelvina). Central overstretching results in a pulsation cystocele with passing of the rugae vaginalis and preserved longitudinal sulci (**Figure 1**). This is more often observed in older patients. In case of lateral tear off of the vagina (uni- or bilateral) from the arcus tendineus fasciae pelvis, a traction cystocele with preserved rugae is found [9]. This defect often occurs after birth trauma and is also found in younger women. Combination of both are common. This disorder can cause urinary incontinence and/or bladder voiding dysfunction. Level-III-Defects are one of the most common reasons for stress incontinence, because of the missing lateral fixation of the urethra [8].

4.1.2 Descensus of the apical compartment

A descensus of the apical compartment (defect in Level I) leads to a uterine prolapse or vaginal stump descensus (after hysterectomy, **Figure 2**). Main cause is the overstretching of the ligaments holding the uterus, in particular the sacrouterine ligament. Depending on the degree of prolapse, one speaks of partial prolapse (the cervix

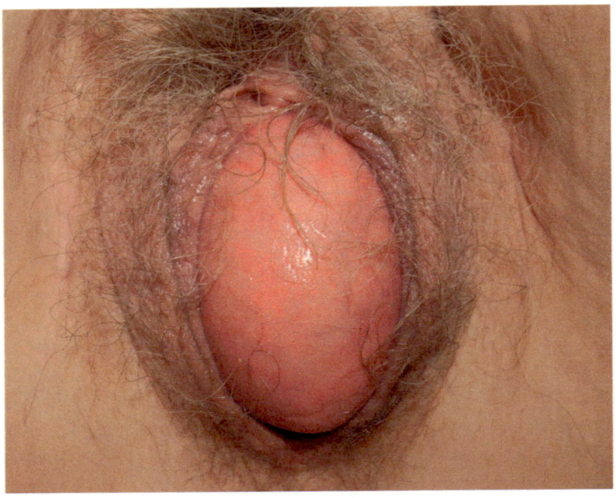

Figure 1.
Pulsation cystocele, stadium 2. With kind permission of Dr. Christian Fünfgeld, all rights reserved.

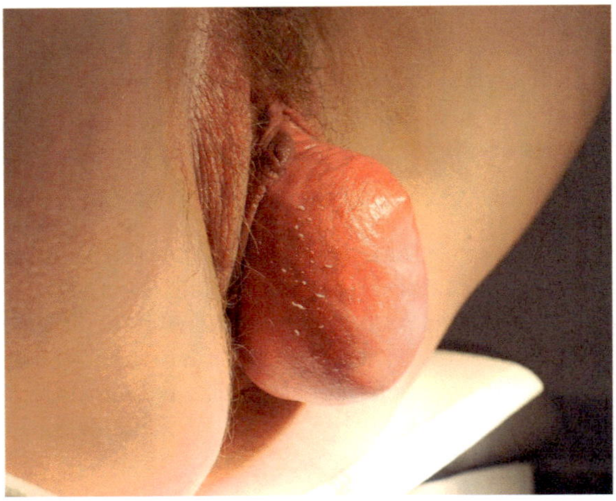

Figure 2.
Vaginal stump prolapse. With kind permission of Dr. Christian Fünfgeld, all rights reserved.

protrudes up to the introitus), prolapse (the cervix protrudes to the introitus or further) or total prolapse with a inversion of the vagina (**Figure 2**). Descensus of the apical compartment is usually less problematic, as it only becomes symptomatic when the prolapse reaches to the introitus or further (**Figure 3**) [9].

4.1.3 Descensus of the posterior compartment

A descensus of the posterior compartment leads to a recto- or enterocele (**Figure 4**). A defect of the rectovaginal septum leads to a protrusion of the vaginal posterior wall. This leads to ventral displacement of the rectum, whose circumference usually increases, which, in turn, can cause defecation disorder. Especially for the diagnosis of rectocele, letting the patient squeeze is crucial. Herniation of the small intestine into the pelvis between the rectum and vagina then leads to an enterocele, which occurs more often after hysterectomy. Especially when there is a Burch colposuspension performed additionally to a hysterectomy, the risk for developing an enterocele increases [9].

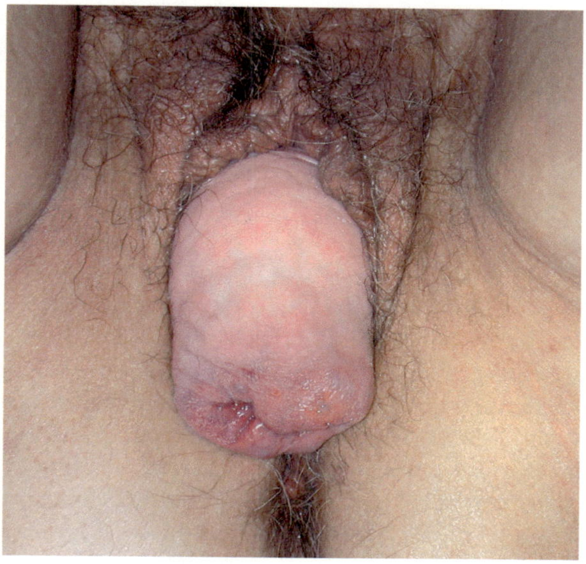

Figure 3.
Uterine prolapse, stadium 3. With kind permission of Dr. Christian Fünfgeld, all rights reserved.

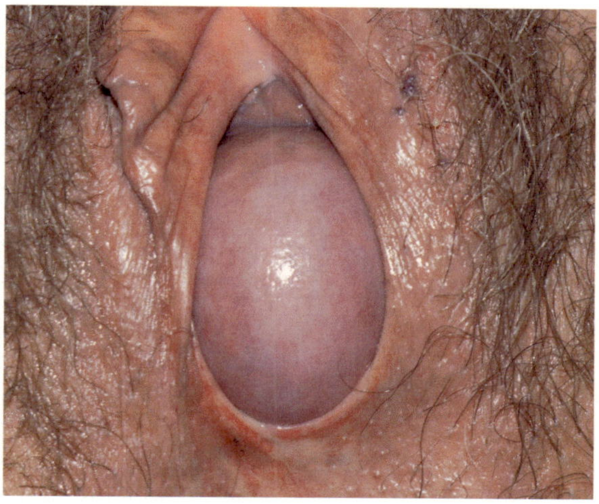

Figure 4.
Rectocele, stadium 4. With kind permission of Dr. Christian Fünfgeld, all rights reserved.

4.2 Urinary incontinence

Urinary incontinence can be divided into two main groups- stress incontinence and urgency incontinence. Stress incontinence occurs when the pelvic floor is exposed to stress, for example during coughing, laughing or during physical exertion. In can be further divided into degrees, depending on the situation when loss of urine occurs.

- I—loss of urine when coughing, sneezing or laughing
- II—loss of urine when moving, for example when getting up, during sports
- III—loss of urine without moving, when lying

Urgency incontinence describes the loss of urine combined with a sudden urge to urinate. A special form of urgency incontinence is the overactive bladder syndrome, which is defined as urge to urinate, which can or cannot be accompanied by urge incontinence, usually escorted by a high micturition interval and nocturia. Stress and urgency often occur together [10].

5. Symptoms

Symptoms of pelvic floor disorders usually develop gradually and slowly over time. Unfortunately, symptoms associated with pelvic floor disorders are still a taboo and women often take a long time before opening up to their gynecologist and to seek help for their condition. Problems which are then reported are primarily symptoms of prolapse (Feeling of something coming out of the vagina, downward pressure, pain), urinary or fecal incontinence or bladder voiding dysfunction. The latter often leads to recurrent UTIs. Both stress and urge incontinence can occur as common symptoms of prolapse, whilst anal incontinence is rather rare. Instead, in the context of a rectocele, defecation disorders occur more frequently, which are often interpreted by patients as constipation [9].

These symptoms have a high impact on patients` everyday life. Incontinence can lead to avoiding daily social activities, while many patients also avoid drinking enough fluids, in order to avoid the loss of urine. Using incontinence pads also means a financial burden for the women affected. Patients suffering from prolapse often avoid sexual intercourse, because of feeling ashamed, while some even experience painful intercourse. Pelvic floor disorder can have a huge impact on a woman's social, emotional, sexual, physical and financial well-being. Addressing the patient actively and asking about pelvic floor disorder symptoms can be helpful.

6. Diagnostics

At the beginning, a detailed medical history should be taken regarding the complaints, previous births with complications and previous therapy attempts or operations. This should include evaluating where the patient is most distressed and which symptoms are perceived to be the most severe. Medical history should include questions regarding urinary incontinence, bladder voiding dysfunction, anal incontinence, defecation disorders and problems regarding sexuality. Using a questionnaire for evaluating medical history can help to get a first overview on the most urgent sufferings and can help to standardize and compare different group of patients. The most important tool for the diagnosis of pelvic floor disorders is the clinical examination. During the vaginal examination with two separate specula, all three compartments can be assessed at rest, during elevation and during pressing and should be classified according to the ICS/IUGA-classification [8]. A clinical distinction can also already be made between a pulsation cystocele (rugae vaginalis passed) and a traction cystocele (rugae preserved). While protrusion of the posterior vaginal wall is mostly well visible, a distinction between a rectocele or a enterocele needs additional diagnostic measures. Uterine prolapse or vaginal stump descensus is also easy to assess in clinical examination. To assess pelvic floor contractility and width of the genital hiatus, vaginal palpation should follow after speculum examination. A rectal examination with assessment of the sphincter resting tone and contractility should also be carried out routinely. Subsequently, vaginal ultrasound to evaluate the anatomy of the urethra and the bladder, but also their position and mobility, should be carried out. Is also allows direct imaging of alloplastic implant, if present. Ultrasound can also be used to distinguish between recto- and enterocele. In addition, endoanal ultrasonography can be used to assess the sphincter ani and its damage. With these easily accessible examination technique, most patients with pelvic floor disorders can be diagnosed sufficiently [8]. For complex cases, additional examination can be carried out. These can be a dynamic MRI or a defecography for anal incontinence or urodynamic examinations for urine incontinence, including uroflowmetry, cystometrogram, pressure flow study and urethral pressure profile. A cystoscopy may be helpful for some issues and an interdisciplinary presentation of the patient involving urology, proctology, surgery, and possibly neurology may still be considered. Sometimes, patients with drastic anatomical changes do not experience as many symptoms as patients who objectively only have minor clinical findings. Here, particularly in the case of dramatically described symptoms, it can be helpful to use a drinking and micturition log or a stool diary to assess and objectify the dysfunction [8].

7. Therapy

7.1 Conservative therapy

Without wanting to diminish the suffering of patients, pelvic floor disorders are of course not life-threatening conditions. Therefore, conservative therapy measures should first be offered and tried by the patient before surgical therapy. Depending on which symptom is the most prominent, various conservative methods are available. When a patient is suffering from stress urinary incontinence, pelvic floor training can improve functionality. The pelvic floor training should be supervised by a physiotherapist specialized in this field and can be supported by biofeedback or electrostimulation. Patients suffering from an overactive bladder and urge incontinence can benefit from bladder conditioning through behavioral training (toilet training) and anticholinergic therapy [9]. Anticholinergic medication should be tried for at least 3 months and the patient should be informed about possible side effects such as dry mouth or constipation. Other pharmacotherapy options are alpha-adrenoreceptor blockers for bladder voiding dysfunction and beta3-adrenoreceptor agonists like Mirabegron for overavtive bladder syndrome. A micturition diary can help to objectify whether medication is working or not. After menopause, incontinence symptoms can be improved by the use of local vaginal estrogens. All conservative measures should always be accompanied by lifestyle modifications like weight loss, nicotine abstinence and reducing caffeine intake, which can also optimize surgical outcome, if surgical therapy is planned next. Use of different types of pessaries can be useful to treat uterus prolapse and cystoceles, if tolerated by the patient, while treatment of rectoceles with a pessary is more complicated. There are different sizes and types of pessaries available, which can be individually customized. Often, sieve bowl pessaries are more effective in a cystocele and cube pessaries are better in descensus uteri or rectocele. It is necessary to try different pessaries to find which one gives the patient the most relief and holds best under movement without dislocating. The patient should be trained to change the pessary independently to lower the risk for infections and injuries. Especially in younger patients whose family planning has not yet been completed, pessary therapy should be preferred to surgical therapy. This also applies to older, multimorbid patients [8]. Regarding anal incontinence, stool thickening by appropriate nutrition or by medication (e.g. loperamide) can improve quality of life. Defecation disorder can be treated with dietary options or through laxatives. Conservative therapy should always be performed in consultation with the patient and reviewed regularly. If necessary, a change to surgical therapy may be required if there is insufficient improvement or compliance. Moreover, there may be some patients who are not willing to try conservative therapy and immediately demand a permanent solution, which can only be achieved by surgery [9].

7.2 Surgical therapy

The therapy should be individually optimized to provide an optimal solution for each individual patient. Generally, the indication for pelvic floor surgery is elective. Therefore, the degree of suffering of the affected person is always decisive for the indication of a surgical intervention. Asymptomatic findings of descensus should not be operated on. If surgery is indicated, the goal is usually reconstruction of the anatomic situation. However, the patient desires a restitution of function and thus an elimination of symptoms. Unfortunately, even a successful anatomical reconstruction cannot always guarantee a cure of the symptoms. It is imperative to inform the patients about this. In particular, the occurrence of de novo incontinence should be mentioned. Positional changes can often be corrected effectively, in contrast to muscle or nerve damage. However, since the often weak connective tissue remains unchanged, there is a considerable risk of recurrence. This should also be discussed with the patient. In addition, it should be clarified with the patient what degree of stability she expects and needs from the operation [9].

The spectrum of surgical possibilities has expanded considerably in the last three decades. Previously, for over 100 years, vaginal hysterectomy with anterior and posterior colporrhaphy was the standard gynecologic procedure for any form of cystocele, uterine descensus, or rectocele. This usually can correct descensus satisfactorily. However, the recurrence rate is relatively high and amounts to 37% after 12 months for anterior colporrhaphy according to the current guideline for genital descensus [11]. Therefore, analogous to hernia surgery, attempts have been made to improve long-term stability by implanting alloplastic meshes and ligaments. The anatomical recurrence rate was significantly lower after implantation of alloplastic material (7%) [12]. In the subjective assessment, the difference is smaller. Due to a frequent lack of experience in surgeons and a generous use of the initially too small-pored and too heavy-weighted meshes, there have been considerable adverse events and complications, so that now, especially in Anglo-Saxon countries, alloplastic meshes and tapes are banned or can only be used under strict regulations [13]. The German Working Group for Urogynecology and Pelvic Floor Surgery (AGUB) has a more differentiated view and considers the use of these materials with an appropriate indication in the case of recurrent prolapse, very weak connective tissue or severe descensus with a high risk of recurrence in the hands of a urogynecologically specialized surgeon as justified and often necessary [9]. The complication rate could be significantly reduced with the further development of materials and the optimization of the surgical technique. In addition to the vaginal approach, the abdominal/laparoscopic approach has also gained importance in recent years. Today, hysterectomy is mostly only part of a descensus operation if there is a corresponding additional indication.

7.3 Surgical therapy: rectocele

Only after exhausting the conservative methods should surgical therapy of a rectocele be considered. In gynecology, a rectocele is usually treated with a posterior vaginoplasty. On closer inspection, this is not a consistent surgical procedure. Under this term, the posterior colporrhaphia, the pelviperineoplasty, a fascia-specific repair or a median fascia lift are summarized- in each case with or without levatorplasty or bulbospongiosus lift, which differ considerably in the structures that are "lifted". For stabilization, an alloplastic mesh can also be implanted. However, the results between simple posterior plastic and mesh-supported posterior plastic differ less than with the anterior plastic. Biological patches can be also used, but showed worse results [11].

A transanal or transperineal operation, a Stapled Trans Anal Rectal Resection (STARR) or a laparoscopic or open resection rectopexy are the portfolio of a coloproctological surgeon. Studies that would provide valid data comparing the different gynecological and surgical techniques are still not available. In surgical studies, the change in the stool diary is usually used as a success parameter. The gynecological studies mostly assess the anatomical success of the posterior vaginal wall without recording the improvement in quality of life.

In the current German gynecological guideline on descensor surgery, after extensive literature research on rectocele correction, the following results were found [7]:

Success rates (follow-up time > 12 months):

- posterior vaginoplasty with autologous tissue: median fascia lift: 82–93%
- posterior vaginoplasty with autologous tissue: defect-specific correction: 56–91%
- posterior vaginoplasty with autologous tissue and levator suture: 76–96%
- surgeries using non-resorbable synthetic meshes: 78–100%

Alloplastic materials are definitely indicated for recurrent rectoceles, pronounced findings, high risk of recurrence and accompanying enteroceles that are otherwise often difficult to correct. Since there is little self-tissue in the upper posterior part of the vagina to stabilize a rectocele, it can sometimes be difficult to correct the rectocele without using an alloplastic mesh and without causing dyspareunia through conventional colporrhaphy. Reconstruction of the rectovaginal septum alone to reduce the posterior vaginal wall without reducing the circumference of the rectum, which is usually too large, increases the risk of intussusception. If intussusception or rectal prolapse is more pronounced preoperatively, an interdisciplinary gynecological and coloproctological investigation should be carried out. Coloproctological surgery procedures are often more suitable here. Less pronounced intussusceptions can be treated via transanal access. If there is a posterior wall prolapse combined with a rectocele and intussusception or anal prolapse, a two-stage surgical concept can be useful [8].

First, a gynecological reconstruction is carried out and then, if the result is functionally unsatisfactory, a secondary coloproctological operation can be carried out- or vice versa. Ultimately, when planning therapy, focus should be on restoring quality of life by reducing symptoms.

7.4 Surgical therapy: enterocele

An enterocele is a challenge for surgical therapy. Since an enterocele rarely occurs isolated, correction is carried out in combination with interventions to repair a cystocele, rectocele or descent of the vaginal stump or uterus. In case of vaginal access, an opening and resection of the enterocele hernial sac with a subsequent "high peritonealization" is carried out. An alloplastic mesh can be used to stabilize the upper part of the posterior vagina, as there is usually little autologous tissue available here [8].

7.5 Surgical therapy: cystocele and descent of vaginal stump or uterus

The therapy of the cystocele is complex. Vaginal, abdominal and laparoscopic approaches are possible. The choice of the procedure ultimately also depends on the patient's wishes and on whether and which other compartments are affected by a descent.

The German Deszensus guideline confirms that anterior vaginoplasty is a good option in patients who have not previously been operated on, especially with simultaneous apical fixation [9]. According to the Cochrane Review of 2016 and other systematic reviews, mesh augmentation in the anterior compartment is superior to surgery with autologous tissue, i.e. anterior vaginoplasty [12]. A wide variety of meshes are available on the market. Which is possibly better than another cannot be described with the available data, since no comparative studies are available. However, patients did not benefit from using biological materials [11].

In the past, hysterectomy was usually a key part of a descensus-, but also often of incontinence surgery. Vaginal hysterectomy with anterior and posterior colporrhaphy was the most frequently chosen operation. If incontinence was in the foreground or a vaginal approach seemed impossible, abdominal hysterectomy with retropubic colposuspension (with several procedures as according to Marshall-Marchetti-Kranz, Hirsch, Burch, Stanton, Cowan etc.) can be considered. With the introduction of alloplastic implants and the triumph of laparoscopy, the spectrum expanded considerably. The possibility of combining the procedures in different ways makes it increasingly difficult for the surgeon to select the correct procedure [11].

For primary surgery of a cystocele, especially if there is a central defect (pulsation cystocele), conventional anterior colporrhaphy with median fascia lift is still the most suitable procedure. According to the German Deszensus guidelines, however, if there are pronounced stages of prolapse or the desire for improved stability, a primary mesh implantation can be considered. This also applies to patients with a high surgical risk who want to avoid another operation for a relapse. In the case of recurrence of the cystocele, stabilization by using a mesh is recommended. It becomes more difficult with paravaginal defects (traction cystocele). In conventional surgery, there is only the paravaginal repair according to Richardson with attachment of the endopelvic fascia to the tendon arch, which can usually be done through retropubic access, but also vaginally. However, the success rates of this procedure were not convincing. The reason for this is the lack of stabilization of the apex (level 1) and the upper third of the vagina. Still, with increasing use of sacrocolopexy, paravaginal repair is gaining in importance. The stability is achieved by fixation of the apex (cervix or vaginal end) by the mesh fixed on the sacrum/promontory. The correction of the cystocele, which is not always sufficient, can be improved by lateral fixation. This combination is more complex, but is preferable to a vaginal mesh, especially for younger patients. For older patients with a pronounced lateral defect, treatment with a vaginal mesh-supported plastic is very effective [11]. Whereas in the past the focus was on treating cystoceles and rectoceles, the focus of the descensus surgery has nowadays shifted towards stabilization in level 1. Fixing the cervix or the vaginal stump after hysterectomy brings better results, not only for level 1, but also for the cystocele. A cystocele correction with or without mesh shows fewer recurrences if the apex is fixed at the same time. Several methods are available today for this purpose. Sacrospinal fixation of the vaginal stump (several modifications according to Amreich and Richter) has become established for the vaginal access. Today, this procedure is also performed while preserving the uterus with fixation of the cervix to the sacrospinal ligament. The sacrospinal fixation in the original technique or with a band system can be performed with the uterus in place or with a hysterectomy primarily or in the event of a relapse. It can be easily combined with conventional colporrhaphy. The abdominal or laparoscopic approach has proven to be a further approach for level 1 fixation [11].

After being informed by the surgeon, the patient has the right to participate in the choice of the surgical procedure. Some want good stability, so that a mesh can be implanted, while others do not want one for fear of alloplastic implants. Likewise, many strictly reject a hysterectomy, others wish it because of existing pathology. The indication is becoming more and more complex due to the multitude of options available. The advantage, however, is that you can offer an operation concept that is individually tailored to the patient and the present findings [11].

7.6 Surgical therapy: urinary incontinence

Surgical therapy is highly effective in stress incontinence with placement of mid-urethral slings being the first line option. Retropubic and transobturator pathways are possible. The treatment of urgency incontinence is more complex. Neuromodulation is one possibility, if pharmacotherapy is not effective for urgency incontinence. Another possible treatment option is the intravesical injection of botulinumtoxin A, which usually lasts up to 12 months and can be repeated, if necessary [10].

8. Prevention

The prevention of anorectal dysfunction, but also of descensus and urinary incontinence, begins at the latest after a woman has given birth. Training the pelvic floor muscles, weight optimization, avoiding constipation, learning a pelvic floor-friendly carrying technique and nicotine abstinence can reduce the risk for developing pelvic floor disorders. Postmenopausal, local vaginal application of estriol has proliferating effects on the vaginal, urethral and bladder epithelia and improves blood flow in the urethral area. Hereby, descensus can also be prevented or delayed [8].

Author details

Isabell Link* and Christian Fünfgeld
Department of Gynecology and Obstetrics, Clinic Tettnang, Germany

*Address all correspondence to: isabell.link@gmx.de

References

[1] Samuelsson EC, Victor FT, Tibblin G, Svärdsudd KF. Signs of genital prolapse in a Swedish population of women 20 to 59 years of age and possible related factors. American Journal of Obstetrics and Gynecology. 1999;**180**:299-305

[2] Hannestad YS, Rortveit G, Sandvik H, et al. A community-based epidemiological survey of female urinary incontinence: The Norwegian EPINCONTStudy. Journal of Clinical Epidemiology. 2000;**53**:1150-1157

[3] Nygaard I, Barber MD, Burgio KL, et al. Prevalence of symptomatic pelvic floor disorders in US women. JAMA. 2008;**300**:1311

[4] Fialkow MF, Newton KM, Lentz GM, Weiss NS. Lifetime risk of surgical management for pelvic organ prolapse or urinary incontinence. International Urogynecology Journal Pelvic Floor Dysfunction. 2008;**19**:437-433

[5] Olsen AL, Smith VJ, Bergstrom JO, Colling JC, Clark AL. Epidemiology of surgically managed pelvic organ prolapse and urinary incontinence. Obstetrics and Gynecology. 1997; **89**:501-506

[6] Gyhagen M, Bullarbo M, Nielsen TF, et al. The prevalence of urinary incontinence 20 years after childbirth: A national cohort study in singleton primiparae after vaginal or caesarean delivery. International Journal of Obstetrics and Gynaecology. 2013; **120**(2):144-151

[7] AWMF online: Leitlinienreport zur S2e-Leitlinie 015/006: Diagnostik und Therapie des weiblichen Deszensus genitalis. Available from: www.awmf.org/uploads/tx_szleitlinien/015-006m_S2e_Descensus_genitalis-Diagnostik-Therapie_2016-05.pdf.Zugriff06.09.02021

[8] Fünfgeld C. 18. Gynäkologie in der Koloproktologie. In: Herold A, Schiedeck T, editors. Manual der Koloproktologie. Bd. 1 ed. Berlin, Boston: De Gruyter; 2019. pp. S259-S270.DOI:10.1515/9783110614442-018

[9] Fünfgeld C. Diagnostik und Therapie der weiblichen Beckenbodeninsuffizienz. In: coloproctology. Medizin: Springer; 2020. DOI: 10.1007/s00053020-00438-9

[10] Aoki Y, Brown HW, Brubaker L, Cornu JN, Daly JO, Cartwright R. Urinary incontinence in women. Nature Reviews Disease Primers. 2017;**16**(3): 17097. DOI: 10.1038/nrdp.2017.42

[11] Fünfgeld C, Niesel A, editors. Operationstechniken in der Urogynäkologie bei Deszensus und Harninkontinenz. UNI-MED Verlag AG: Bremen-London-Boston; 2020

[12] Maher C, Feiner B, Baessler K, Christmann-Schmid C, Haya N, Marjoribanks J. Transvaginal mesh or grafts compared with native tissue repair for vaginal prolapse. Cochrane Database of Systematic Reviews. 2016;**2**(2):CD012079. Published 2016 Feb 9. DOI: 10.1002/14651858.CD012079

[13] Niesel A, Gabriel B, Tunn R, Fünfgeld C. Alloplastische implantate: Internationale diskussionund regelungen. Frauenarzt. 2019;**60**(5): 1997-2002

Chapter 2

Pelvic Floor Muscle Activity in Relation to Body Position and Breath

Monika Sorfova and Eva Tlapakova

Abstract

The aim of this work was to analyse pelvic floor muscle activity by intravaginal perineometry. We focused on the increase caused by phasic muscular activity, which, on a short term basis, rises above the basal tonic activity. The functional relationships to postural and respiratory function have been confirmed by only a few studies. Therefore, we monitored this functional connection. We confirmed a statistically significant increase in pelvic floor muscle activity at deep breathing compared to calm breathing (in other words at different breathing intensity) in the same position (lying, standing). Our measurements also showed that the phasic activity of pelvic floor muscles in deep breathing is statistically significantly higher than activity after a minute-long run on the treadmill. Cough is a specific situation, whose short-term increase in pelvic floor muscle activity clearly exceeds all other monitored situations.

Keywords: pelvic floor muscle, breathing, perineometer, body position

1. Introduction

In 1948, Dr. Kegel [1] developed an intravaginal device, a perineometer, for assessing pelvic floor muscle strength. A pressure vaginal probe was connected to a manometer to measure the intravaginal pressure induced by the contraction of the pelvic floor muscles in mmHg. Since then, pressure probes of various shapes and technical properties have been developed [2, 3]. One type of instrument used under standard conditions with a well-guided protocol is very useful for both objectifying the diagnostics and assessing the effect of therapy [4].

The pelvic floor performs two types of activities - tonic and phasic [5, 6], as confirmed by the Deindl study [7]. According to Frawley [3], manometric measurement is one of the most widespread and the advantage is that it allows the measurement of muscle contraction both when lying and standing. This advantage is that incontinence occurs especially in upright positions and therefore examination in these positions will give us information with a higher informative value. It appears that the resting pressure measurement (tonic pressure) is not as reliable in standing (ICC 0.29) and sitting position as in lying (ICC 0.77). Measurement of the pressure of phasic compression of pelvic floor muscle shows good ICC confidence of 0.91 to 0.95 in all body positions [3].

Junginger et al. [8] controlled the decline of the uterine throat and the descent of pelvic organs while increasing intraabdominal pressure, which was prevented by joint activity of the pelvic floor muscles and the transversus abdominis muscles. Iacobellis et al. also conducted a detailed study of the risk of organ descent by MR [9]. Comparing the lying and sitting situation, the difference proved to be statistically significant. This suggests that examination in lying position can underestimate the existing descent of organs.

Bø et al. [10] also ask the question whether a usual manometric examination of the pelvic floor in a lying position is sufficient or whether it is more appropriate to perform examination in a standing position. For standing persons, it has been proved that the pressure increase during will-induced contraction and dwell time have not changed, only the minimum value (tonic contraction) when standing has increased.

The pelvic floor is given responsibility for the continence of urine, stool and the supporting function of the pelvic organs. The connection between the function of the pelvic floor and respiration is rarely considered. Therefore, we wanted to contribute to the knowledge of these connections. In addition, we were interested in the difference in the functional context in the position of the body in a standing and lying position. We performed the measurements even after a minute-long run, which triggered the spontaneous deep breathing process.

2. Methods

During the actual measurement, the person was placed on the examination bed in a position with the legs bent and with the feet propped up, and a condom-protected perionometer probe was inserted. Subsequently, a trained therapist gave verbal instructions and checked the performance. In order to ensure all the required conditions and to eventually register an individual proband response, a second specialist therapist was present during the testing, as recommended by Bø [10], to ensure standardisation of the examination. The individual test manoeuvres were based on a commonly performed PERFECT SCALE examination, which is primarily designed for palpation vaginal examination, but allows the same procedure to be performed via a pressure probe and thus objectifying the results [11].

Maximum contraction and endurance at this level were tested for 10 seconds with subsequent relaxation. In addition, the test subject was asked to repeat maximum contraction and release with a duration of five seconds per phase. Subsequently, a similar situation was tested, but with a shorter duration of individual phases - 1 s contraction and 1 s relaxation. Finally, the person was asked to cough, which was repeated three times. See **Figure 1**.

The second observed phenomenon was the effect of respiration, each examination lasted one minute. We compared the activity of pelvic floor muscles with calm and deep breathing without will-induced activation of pelvic floor muscles. During deep breathing, the proband was instructed to take several deeper inhalations (3 s) and exhalations (6 s). Inhale was done through the nose, exhale through the mouth using the "S" spoken throughout the exhalation. Then the proband switched to the KETTLER TRACK 3 treadmill with the probe installed and ran for a minute on this belt with a 0% slope, i.e. flat and at a speed of 5 km/h. Subsequently, we observed changes in pelvic floor muscle pressures during spontaneous breathing after a minute of running on a treadmill.

To this measurement project were involved 10 women. Their average age was 38 years (range 25–47 years), average height 166.8 cm (range 159–178 cm), average weight 66.9 kg (range 50–85 kg), average BMI 23.9 kg/m^2 (range 19.0–29.8 kg/m^2). There were no births in 3 women, one birth was performed by one woman, two and

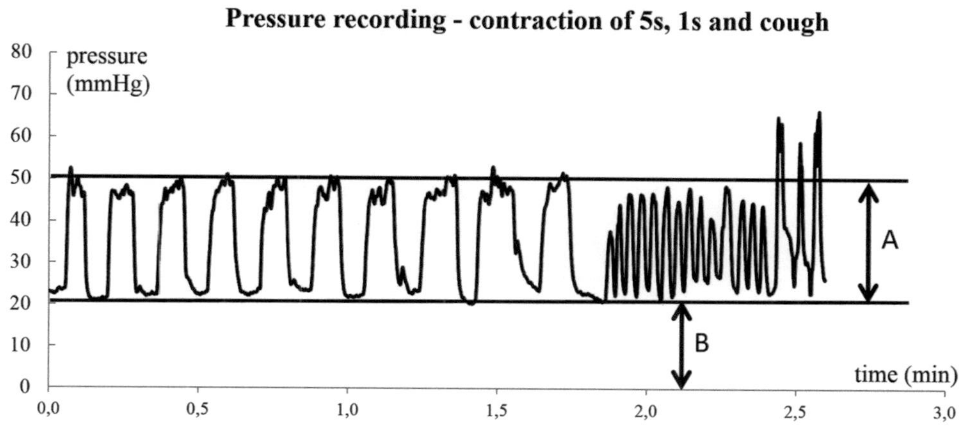

Figure 1.
Subtraction of parameters from measured data - tonic basis of muscle activity (value B). Increase in pressure by A-value in phasic muscular activity (here at the therapist's instruction to repeat will-induced contraction of 5 s and 1 s of pelvic floor muscles and in coughing - three reps).

three births each by two women, and only one woman had 4 births. Only probands who excluded respiratory diseases, abdominal or gynaecological operations, except births, lumbar spine pain, were included in the measurement. No proband is an active athlete.

All statistical calculations were performed using the software OriginPro 8.5.1 (http://www.originlab.com/Origin). T-tests were used to test hypotheses to determine if there was a significant difference between the averages of the two groups of measurements under the given test conditions. Spearman's rank correlation coefficients were calculated to evaluate the associations between variables. The significant at an alpha level of 0.025 (at least) or it is specified in the Results chapter for the specific situations.

3. Results

The achieved increase in perionatal pressure (amplitude) was to be maintained for 10 seconds. This was ideally achieved by one person only. Six persons experienced a gradual decrease in the achieved maximum value by an average of 45% (values 31 to 78%).

As expected, a statistically significant difference can be demonstrated for the tonic activity of the pelvic floor muscles in the lying and standing positions, on average the standing values are 7.5 to 10 mm Hg higher (**Figure 2**). This result fully corresponds to the research of Bø et al. (Bø & Finckenhagen, 2003).

The results are not conclusive for the phasic activity, the amplitude increased statistically significantly only for cough (**Table 1**). The amplitudes of the 1 s and 5 s tests were comparable. Basal tonic pressure values - especially the critically low values observed in three individuals - do not condition the low values achieved in short-term amplitudes.

In the test of pelvic floor muscles reaction to cough, we investigate reflex functions in contrast to will-induced contractions in previous tests (5 s and 1 s). In this case, we clearly find higher amplitudes of contractions in cough, on average, the values are doubled, for one person, the cough pressure is up to 10 times the values of the person's deliberately induced amplitude. The t-test values are statistically significant when comparing cough with all will-induced activities at a significance level of 0.001. As expected, the difference in tonic muscle activity was not detected (**Figure 2**).

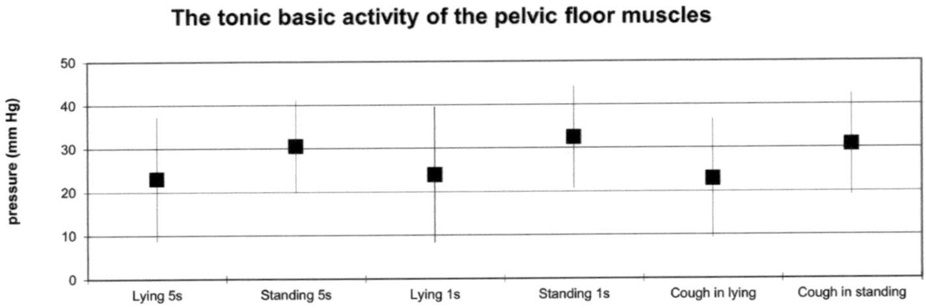

Figure 2.
The tonic pelvic floor muscles activity in specific body position (arithmetic means and determinative deviations).

Comparison lying-standing body position				
	Evaluated			
	Phasic activity		*Tonic activity*	
	t-test	Significance level	t-test	Significance level
Cough	2,271	0,025	3,995	0,002
Calm breathing	3,554	0,003	5,275	0
Deep breathing	3,636	0,003	4,531	0,001

Table 1.
The t-test values significancy - comparing cough with breathing activities fulfilling experimenter's instruction.

In an effort to understand more deeply the above-described morphological-functional interconnections and behaviour of the system during the will-induced and reflexive (or spontaneous) changes, we extended the tested functional situations. We were wondering what the functional response to deepened breathing would be, which we invoke not spontaneously but based on the instructions of the therapist. In addition, a short-term anaerobic load lasting several tens of seconds was chosen.

A statistically significant increase in pelvic floor muscle activity during deep breathing was demonstrated. Comparing this activity with consciously induced deep breathing while standing, with the spontaneous breathing caused by the previous running activity can be considered a very interesting result (**Figure 3**). Phasic activity of pelvic floor muscles in deep breathing is statistically significantly higher than that measured in deepened breath after physical exercise of the tested person for a minute of running on the treadmill.

The statistical comparison shows that the increase in the pelvic floor muscular phasic pressure due to cough differs significantly in all the situations tested, i.e. it differs in relation to the position (lying, standing) and to three types of breathing (quiet, deep, after running) (**Figure 4** and **Table 2**).

While in deep breathing we find large variations of values, in spontaneous breath after a minute-run, the values are scattered minimally, similarly to calm breath in both monitored positions, which we consider an interesting result.

If we monitor the variability of the observed values within the measured group, we can see that while in deep breathing we find large variations of the values of physical pressure increase, in spontaneous breath after a minute run, the values are scattered to a minimum extent, similarly to calm breath. Everything applies to both standing and lying position (**Figure 4**).

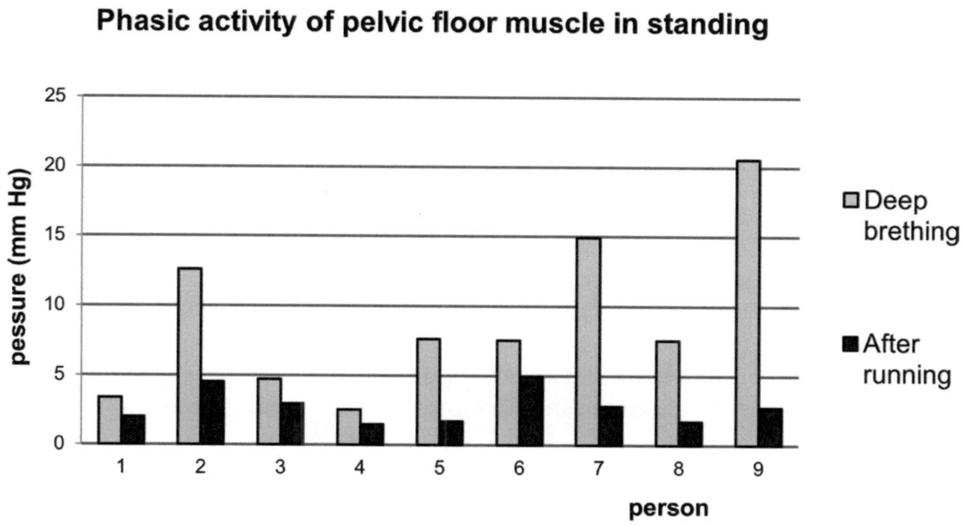

Figure 3.
Phasic muscle activity in deep breathing after running and fulfilling experimenter's instruction.

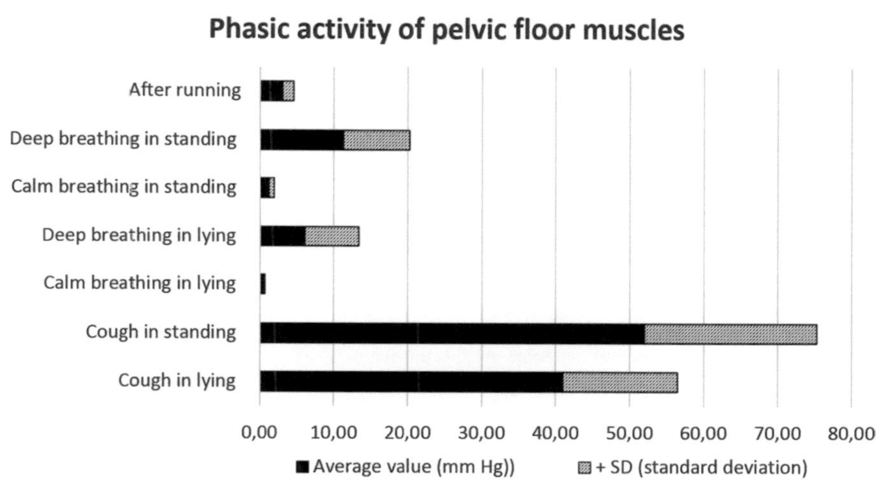

Figure 4.
Values of arithmetic means and determinative deviations for observed situations.

Comparison calm and deep breathing		
Evaluated is phasic muscle activity		
	t-test	**Significance level**
Lying - calm vs. deep breathing	−2,443	0,019
Standing - calm vs. deep breathing	−3,636	0,003
Standing - calm vs. after running	−3,563	0,003
Standing – deep vs. after running	3,209	0,005

Table 2.
Comparison calm and deep breathing and situation after a minute run.

4. Discussion

The aim of our work was to assess how the degree of functional involvement of the pelvic floor changes based on breathing of the tested person, depending on the position of the body in an upright position or lying down.

Our results showed statistically significant differences in tonic activity of pelvic floor muscles in lying and standing position. At the same time, however, we found in the initial study that the will-induced - that is, the phasic muscular contractions of the pelvic floor muscles are not different when comparing measurements taken while standing or lying down (**Table 3**). In other words, the amplitude increase (the value of the short-term pressure increase referred to as phasic action) was approximately the same for both lying and standing position, only when lying down there was a lower level of tonic contraction than when standing (the value of sustained tonic activity).

Only in reflex muscle activity (i.e. cough simulation), differences were detected not only in tonic muscle activity, but also in phasic muscle activity. Thus, it can be argued that this spontaneous response of the system to a cough maintains a tendency to higher amplitudes. This happens both when lying and standing. To evaluate the associations between lying or standing activity, Spearman correlation coefficients were calculated for the same breath type (**Table 4**).

Our results show that the instruction to deepen breathing led to a different increase in the phasic muscular activity of these muscles. Phasic activity of pelvic floor muscles in deep breathing is statistically significantly higher than that measured in deepened breath after physical exercise of the tested person for a minute of running on the treadmill.

Comparison lying-standing body position		
	Evaluated	
Experimenter's instruction	*Phasic activity*	*Tonic activity*
Intertionally contracted	no	yes
Deep breathing	yes	yes
Cough	yes	yes

Table 3.
Comparison of the response of the phasic and tonic activity of the pelvic floor muscles to the experimenter's instruction ("yes" means an increase in standing activity confirmed by mathematical statistics).

Spearman's correlation - lying-standing body position				
	Evaluated			
	Phasic activity		*Tonic activity*	
	Correlation coefficient	**Significance level**	**Correlation coefficient**	**Significance level**
Cough	0,761	0,05	**0,892**	**0,01**
Calm breathing	0,233	no	**0,902**	**0,01**
Deep breathing	**0,86**	**0,01**	**0,914**	**0,01**

Table 4.
Test of the relationship between the increase of tonic and phasic activity of muscles by changing the position of the body.

The functional relationships of postural and respiratory function of the pelvic floor is known. But many clinical procedures rely on only one of these areas. It is more advantageous for the patient to undergo therapy linking the functional influence of the whole respiratory system and the pelvic floor system.

Not only in the direct treatment of pelvic floor dysfunctions, but also in the treatment of widespread low back pain. In routine clinical practice, the pelvic floor, in a patient with back pain, is not examined. If we remove all the pathologies found in the patient - muscle spasms, trigger points, joint blockages, muscle contractions, etc., without treatment of the pelvic floor, the patient will have temporary relief, but the pain will return.

Acknowledgements

The study was supported by SVV 2017-2019-260346 and PROGRES Q41.

Author details

Monika Sorfova* and Eva Tlapakova
Department of Anatomy and Biomechanics, Faculty of Physical Education and Sport, Charles University, Prague, Czech Republic

*Address all correspondence to: sorfova@seznam.cz; sorfova@ftvs.cuni.cz

References

[1] Kegel, A. H. The nonsurgical treatment of genital relaxation; use of the perineometer as an aid in restoring anatomic and functional structure. Ann West Med Surg, 1948; 2(5), s. 213-216. ISSN 0002-9378

[2] Bø, K., Raastad, R., & Finckenhagen, H. B. Does the size of the vaginal probe affect measurement of pelvic floor muscle strength? Acta obstetricia et gynecologica Scandinavica, 2005; 84(2), s. 129-133. ISSN 1600-0412

[3] Frawley, H. C., Galea, M. P., Phillips, B. A., Sherburn, M., & Bø, K. Reliability of pelvic floor muscle strength assessment using different test positions and tools. Neurourology and urodynamics, 2006; 25(3), s. 236-242. ISSN 1520-6777

[4] Rahmani, N., & Mohseni-Bandpei, M. A. Application of perineometer in the assessment of pelvic floor muscle strength and endurance: a reliability study. Journal of bodywork and movement therapies, 2011; 15(2), s. 209-214. ISSN 1360-8592

[5] Sapsford, R. Rehabilitation of pelvic floor muscles utilizing trunk stabilization. Manual therapy, 2004; 9(1), s. 3-12. ISSN 1356-689X

[6] Peschers, U. M., Vodusek, D. B., Fanger, G., Schaer, G. N., Delancey, J. O., & Schuessler, B. Pelvic muscle activity in nulliparous volunteers. Neurourology and urodynamics, 2001; 20(3), s. 269-275. ISSN 1520-6777

[7] Deindl, F., Vodusek, D., Hesse, U., & Schussler, B. Activity patterns of pubococcygeal muscles in nulliparous continent women. British Journal of urology, 1993; 72(1), s. 46-51. ISSN 1464-410X

[8] Junginger, B., Baessler, K., Sapsford, R., & Hodges, P. W. Effect of abdominal and pelvic floor tasks on muscle activity, abdominal pressure and bladder neck. International Urogynecology Journal, 2010; 21(1), 69-77. ISSN 0937-3462

[9] Iacobellis, F., Brillantino, A., Renzi, A., Monaco, L., Serra, N., Feragalli, B., . . . Cappabianca, S. MR Imaging in Diagnosis of Pelvic Floor Descent: Supine versus Sitting Position. Gastroenterology Research and Practice. 2016; ISSN 1687-6121

[10] Bø, K., & Finckenhagen, H. B. Is there any difference in measurement of pelvic floor muscle strength in supine and standing position? Acta obstetricia et gynecologica Scandinavica, 2003; 82(12), s. 1120-1124. ISSN 1600-0412.

[11] Laycock, J., & Jerwood, D. Pelvic floor muscle assessment: the PERFECT scheme. Physiotherapy, 2001; 87(12), s. 631-642. ISSN 0031-9406

Chapter 3

Perineal Management and Episiotomy Practice in Chile

Cristhel K. Fagerstrom-Sade, Sara Parada-Ibañez, Marcela M. Gurovich, Esther Ayala-Pérez, Pablo Ortega-Plancic, Jaime Roa-Burgos, Fabián Vasquez-Vergara and Jorge Rodriguez-Suazo

Abstract

Episiotomy is a common intervention used during the second stage of delivery. Current use of this procedure is restricted to certain births due to several complications. Almost all births in Chile are delivered by a gynecologist or a midwife in the public or private health system where episiotomy is performed. The objective of this study is to identify strengths and weakness in aspects of perineal management and episiotomy practice among obstetric health care providers with the purpose of promoting practice assessment and updating skills and competencies. Design: Questionnaire-based-cross-sectional study. Method: Anonymous questionnaire applied to gynecologists and midwives of public and private hospitals, between October and December 2019 using the Instrument designed by Cornet et al. addressing questions such as affiliation, number of births/year, knowledge of anatomy, knowledge of episiotomy, knowledge of perineal tear, competence in perineal repair, and presence of expert in perineal trauma at their unit. Results: 189 surveys responded, 51% from midwives and 37.6% from doctors. 71% of total were trained at their medical or midwifery schools and 69% during postgraduate internships. Episiotomy practice criteria: 19% always in primigravida patients and 14,3% always in premature deliveries. Majority of professionals, 79.4% with less than 100 deliveries a year had incorrect answers about depth or sphincter tear prevention technique. Conclusions: The majority of professionals indicated insufficient training capacities in relation to episiotomy techniques. Undergraduate programs should strength training on this intervention, national guidelines must include routine episiotomy performance in order to unify criteria.

Keywords: episiotomy, episiotomies, midwifery, obstetrics, sphincter injuries, clinical practice, Chile

1. Introduction

In Chile vital statistics and indicators are methodically published by the bureau of vital statistics jointly with the national institute of statistics.

Chile has a mixed health system (public and private) in terms of financing, health insurance, and service delivery. Certified health professionals may work in either system. Midwives assist the vast majority of normal deliveries at the public service and in the private sector they work cooperatively with the gyn-ob.

Since 1982 until 2016 the rate of deliveries assisted by skilled health personnel, obstetricians or midwifes was 99,8% [1]. In 2016 the natality rate was 14,8% with 243.149 live newborns and the population was 18.191.000 inhabitants.

Episiotomy is the most commonly intervention practiced in obstetrics. It is recommended in order to facilitate the second stage of delivery and protect pelvic tissues from lacerations as well as the fetal head. The surgical incision was early described by Fielding (1742), Michaelis (1799) and Braun (1857) and has been widely used since then [2].

The routine practice of episiotomy has resulted in many researchers questioning the very purpose of this procedure as well as its potential benefits. Nowadays it is restricted [3] to certain deliveries because of the complications and long term outcomes such as infection, edema, pain, laceration or tearing into perineal muscles, bleeding, urinary and fecal incontinence and also esthetic defects [4–6].

If mediolateral episiotomy is practiced with an angle further than 45-60 degree it will not attain greater median levator muscle relaxation. When episiotomy is to short usually will not reduce perineal tissue stress and may provide a weak angle for uncontrolled laceration [2, 7], therefore inappropriate techniques hold greater risks of rectal sphincter injuries [8].

Medio-lateral episiotomy may prevent the recurrence of obstetric anal sphincter injuries (OASIS) specially in women with history of anal sphincter tears in previous deliveries [9], fetal macrosomia [10], nulliparity [11], first vaginal delivery with previous cesarean section, and a prolonged second stage of labour [10, 12], though discordant benefits have been reported with this procedure [13].

Even though there has been general agreement about restrictive episiotomy recommendations [14–16], available data demonstrates that professional viewpoints [17, 18], indications and individual patient conditions [19], are up until now associated with a large rate of episiotomies [20–23]. Correct categorization of patients based on profesional abilities and skills [7, 24] as well as risk factors [8] are very important in order to prevent OASIS [25].

Events affecting episiotomy recovery are technique used, incision extension, and third or fourth degree tear after procedure [2].

A British study about midwifery practice describes that concealed anal sphincter tears showed a twofold increment when re-evaluated by a qualified health profesional [26]. Still, only 17% of midwives tend to perform a rectal examination [27].

This study was designed to find out the principal strengths and weakness around birth assistance and determine doctors and Midwives competencies in aspects of perineal management and episiotomy practice in Chile, with the purpose of promoting professional practice assessment and updating skills and competencies.

2. Material and methods

A questionnaire-based-cross-sectional study was conducted. We used an anonymous questionnaire sent by mail to midwives and doctors attending births at one or more public and/or private maternity units in order to identify competencies in aspects of perineal management and episiotomy practice. This study took place between October and December 2019 using the Instrument designed by Cornet et al. [28]. Fourteen close-ended questions were incorporated in relation to: profession, affiliation, number of births/year, evaluation on the knowledge of anatomy, evaluation on the knowledge of episiotomy, evaluation of the knowledge of perineal tear and competence in perineal repair, and presence of expert in perineal trauma in his/her unit. Study criteria included certified Obstetrician-Gynecologists and Midwives currently assisting births either at the public or private health system in Chile.

3. Data collection

Initially a pilot study was applied to 18 midwives and obstetricians working at one public hospital in Santiago, during July 2019. After some question corrections, the anonymous questionnaire was sent by means of social media to certified health professionals who assisted deliveries in Chile between October and December 2019. We convoked 189 respondents.

4. Data analysis

A data base was constructed through an Excel file and data were analyzed through the statistical package STATA version 15.0®. A descriptive assessment was primarily carried out. Categorical variables were described in terms of frequencies and proportions. Chi square test was used to establish relationship between variables. Significance level was 5%.

5. Findings

189 surveys were returned, 97 (51,3%) from midwives and 71 (37,6%) from obstetricians. 11% did not state profession. 57% of respondents attend deliveries exclusively at the public health system, 19% at the private system and 14.3% in both (**Table 1**).

70% of participants were trained in episiotomy practice at their undergraduate schools and 69% at medical internships.

The majority of professionals assisted between 20 and 100 deliveries per year and 2,2% of them assisted 500 or more (**Figure 1**).

Regarding episiotomy criteria, there was no homogeneity in their practice, but it is clear that the majority do not perform this procedure as a sphincter injury prevention technique when risk conditions arise (**Table 2**).

When data is divided by groups, professionals who assist ≤100 deliveries/year had more incorrect answers concerning prevention of deep sphincter or perineal injuries vs. those assisting 100 or more deliveries (79.4%) $p < 0.05$ (**Table 3**).

Entity of work	**N**	**%**
Public hospital	(109)	57.7
Private maternity	(34)	18
Public and private practice	(27)	14.3
Home delivery	(4)	2.1
Not responded	(15)	7.9
Total	189	100

Source: Survey "Diagnosis and management of episiotomies" OASI.

Table 1.
Affiliation.

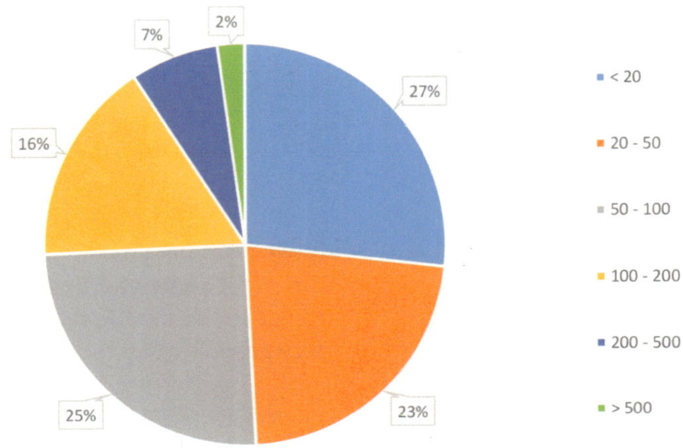

Figure 1.
N° of deliveries attended by the respondents per year.

Condition	Performing episiotomy		Not performing episiotomy	
	N	%	N	%
Primigravida	(36)	19,1	(153)	81
Foetus estimated weight > 3800 grs	(56)	29,6	(133)	70,4
Genitals with edema	(62)	32,8	(127)	67,2
Vulvar varicose veins	(22)	11,6	(167)	88,4
Instrumental delivery	(169)	89,4	(20)	10,6
Preterm birth	(27)	14,3	(162)	85,7
Persistent occiput posterior position	(66)	34,9	(123)	65,1

Source: Survey "Diagnosis and management of episiotomies" OASI.

Table 2.
Criteria for episiotomy utilization.

Condition	<100 deliveries/year		>100 deliveries/year		Total	
	N	%	N	%	N	%
Properly performed	33	63,5	19	36,5	52	28.4
Improperly performed	104	79.4	27	20,6	131	71.5

Source: Survey "Diagnosis and management of episiotomies" OASI Test chi² $p < 0.05$.
**N = 183 respondents to both questions.*

Table 3.
Quality of episiotomy performance/N° of deliveries per year.

According to self-report questionnaire 28.4% of participants perform this procedure in a correct manner.

Routine rectal examination was performed by 53.3% of participants, in contrast 5.4% never practiced this type of digital exam when assessing perineal trauma (**Table 4**). This is an interesting figure considering that professionals assisting <100 deliveries per year performed a higher frequency of rectal examination but no significant difference was demonstrated between groups (**Table 5**).

	n	%
Always	(99)	53.2
Tear or laceration of tissue	(71)	38.2
Rectal sphincter injury (bleeding)	(3)	1.6
Post instrumental delivery	(3)	1.6
Never	(10)	5.4
Total	186	100

Source: Survey "Diagnosis and management of episiotomies" OASI.

Table 4.
Rectal examination criteria.

Delivery N	Always	Tears	Rectal bleeding	Post instrumental delivery	Never
<100 deliveries/year	68	54	3	2	10
	69.4%	14%	100%	100%	100%
>100 deliveries/year	30	16	0	0	0
	30.6%	22,9%	0	0	0
Total	98	70	3	2	10
	100%	100%	100%	100%	100%

Source: Survey "Diagnosis and management of episiotomies" OASI Test chi^2 $p = 0.147$.

Table 5.
Rectal examination/N° of deliveries.

6. Discussion

In 2007 the National Ministry of Public Health published the clinical guide for humanized care during delivery with the main objective of providing access to all pregnant women for appropriate professional assistance during labor and delivery. This assistance guideline draw attention to intra-partum fetal monitoring and other medical interventions such as episiotomy practice. In spite of the recommendation regarding this practice, few other aspects are addressed namely the competencies needed to perform this intervention in order to avoid tears and other adverse events.

Our study demonstrates that near 30% of professionals lack specific episiotomy technique training. This aspect is thoroughly relevant in light of the international evidence assuring that a correct execution of the episiotomy may have significant implications in OASIS. This is the reason why many authors endorse supervised episiotomy practice when training midwives and doctors, with a minimum number of ten before they are permitted to practice [29].

Individual interpretation of whatever particular situation for practicing episiotomies varied among participants of our study. This aspect was also observed in the study published by Gonzalez-Diaz et-al (2015) [30] therefore it is pertinent to regulate this practice and secure a uniform standard technique, also to establish a common and precise criteria with regard to specific clinical situations that need to be approached by this intervention [30].

Although there are post graduate episiotomy training opportunities, still we have professionals that do not perform this technique in a correct fashion.

Considering the international recommendations, when the third stage of labour is completed, a rectal examination should be carried out in order to correctly assess rectal sphincter injuries [30]. We point out that 46,7% of our participants did not perform this recommendation in every delivery, of these, 5.4% revealed they never practiced the examination and 1.6% performed rectal examination solely under rectal bleeding, also 1.6% respondents when assisting an instrumental delivery.

Following data analysis, it becomes evident that there is a need of a particular guideline for health professionals addressing the correct management of perineal injury prevention and a precise practice of episiotomy. Also, there is the need to promote more training at midwifery and medical schools so to secure the precise abilities and practical skills to correctly perform this technique. At the same time, we should broaden the capacity of continuous training courses for these professionals.

7. Conclusion

The majority of health professionals who attend deliveries in Chile work in public hospitals and indicated insufficient training capacities in relation to episiotomy techniques. Criteria for episiotomy utilization is diverse and heterogeneous with no agreement of absolute indications of the procedure.

8. Suggestions

National guideline for health professionals addressing the correct management of perineal injury prevention, precise practice of episiotomy, proper diagnostic techniques of severe perineal trauma and correct perineal repair.

To improve and strengthen specific formal training programs regarding OASI management and major tears repair and implementing simulation training opportunities and expertise during internships and residence years.

To increase research in this and similar topics.

9. Strengths

First study in Chile about episiotomy practice among obstetricians and midwives.

Survey addressing delivery practices along the territory.

Anonymous survey which facilitates honest answers.

10. Limitations of the study

Limited number of participants in order to assess significant differences.

Acknowledgements

We thank doctors and midwives who participated in this survey.

Authors' contributions

All the authors of the manuscript actively participated in the conception, design and analysis of the study and in the writing of the manuscript and approve the manuscript as submitted.

Conflict of interest

None.

Author details

Cristhel K. Fagerstrom-Sade[1*], Sara Parada-Ibañez[2], Marcela M. Gurovich[3], Esther Ayala-Pérez[2], Pablo Ortega-Plancic[4], Jaime Roa-Burgos[4], Fabián Vasquez-Vergara[5] and Jorge Rodriguez-Suazo[2]

1 Universidad del Desarrollo, Santiago, Chile

2 Universidad San Sebastián, Santiago, Chile

3 Universidad Bernardo O'higgins, Santiago, Chile

4 Clínica Dávila, Santiago, Chile

5 INTA, Universidad de Chile, Santiago, Chile

*Address all correspondence to: c.fagerstrom@udd.cl

References

[1] Serie Nacimientos 2000-2015. http://www.deis.cl/wp-content/uploads/2011/05/SerieNacimientos_2000_2015.html. Accessed December 17, 2019.

[2] Muhleman MA, Aly I, Walters A, Topale N, Tubbs RS, Loukas M. To cut or not to cut, that is the question: A review of the anatomy, the technique, risks, and benefits of an episiotomy. Clin Anat. 2017;30(3):362-372. DOI:10.1002/ca.22836

[3] Nassar AH, Visser GHA, Ayres-de-Campos D, et al. FIGO Statement: Restrictive Use Rather than Routine Use of Episiotomy. Int J Gynecol Obstet. 2019;146(1):ijgo.12843. DOI:10.1002/ijgo.12843

[4] Sagi-Dain L, Sagi S. Indications for episiotomy performance – A cross-sectional survey and review of the literature. J Obstet Gynaecol (Lahore). 2016;36(3):361-365. DOI:10.3109/01443615.2015.1065233

[5] Espuña-Pons M, Solans-Domènech M, Sánchez E. Double incontinence in a cohort of nulliparous pregnant women. Neurourol Urodyn. 2012;31(8):1236-1241. DOI:10.1002/nau.22249

[6] Lowder JL, Burrows LJ, Krohn MA, Weber AM. Risk factors for primary and subsequent anal sphincter lacerations: a comparison of cohorts by parity and prior mode of delivery. Am J Obstet Gynecol. 2007;196(4):344.e1-344.e5. DOI:10.1016/J.AJOG.2006.10.893

[7] Andrews V, Thakar R, Sultan AH, Jones PW. Are mediolateral episiotomies actually mediolateral? BJOG An Int J Obstet Gynaecol. 2005;112(8):1156-1158. DOI:10.1111/j.1471-0528.2005.00645.x

[8] P.M. L, T. V, R. C. Systematic overview of outcomes of third and fourth degree perineal tears in episiotomies versus no episiotomies. Int Urogynecol J Pelvic Floor Dysfunct. 2014;25(1):S134-S135. http://www.embase.com/search/results?subaction=viewrecord&from=export&id=L71591620.

[9] Van Bavel J, Ravelli A, Abu-Hanna A, Mol B, Roovers J, De Leeuw J. The effect of a mediolateral episiotomy on the recurrence of obstetrical anal spincter injury (OASI): An analysis of a national registry. Int Urogynecol J. 2018;29. DOI:10.1007/s00192-018-3752-x

[10] van Bavel J, Ravelli ACJ, Abu-Hanna A, Roovers J, Mol BW, de Leeuw JW. Risk factors for the recurrence of obstetrical anal sphincter injury and the role of a mediolateral episiotomy: an analysis of a national registry. BJOG An Int J Obstet Gynaecol. 2020;n/a(n/a). DOI:10.1111/1471-0528.16263

[11] Verghese TS, Champaneria R, Kapoor DS, Latthe PM. Obstetric anal sphincter injuries after episiotomy: Systematic review and meta-analysis. Int Urogynecol J. 2016;27(10):1459-1467. DOI:10.1007/s00192-016-2956-1

[12] Garmi G, Peretz H, Braverman M, Berkovich I, Molnar R, Salim R. Risk factors for obstetric anal sphincter injury: To prolong or to vacuum? Midwifery. 2016;34. DOI:10.1016/j.midw.2015.11.012

[13] Hartmann K, Viswanathan M, Palmieri R, Gartlehner G, Thorp J, Lohr KN. Outcomes of routine episiotomy: A systematic review. J Am Med Assoc. 2005;293(17). DOI:10.1001/jama.293.17.2141

[14] American College of Obstetricians-Gynecologists. ACOG Practice Bulletin. Episiotomy. Clinical Management Guidelines for

Obstetrician-Gynecologists. Number 71, April 2006. Obstet Gynecol. 2006;107(4):957-962. http://www.ncbi.nlm.nih.gov/pubmed/16582142. Accessed January 6, 2020.

[15] Routine vs selective episiotomy: a randomised controlled trial. Lancet. 1993;342(8886-8887):1517-1518. DOI:10.1016/S0140-6736(05)80085-6

[16] Koskas M, Caillod A-L, Fauconnier A, Bader G. Impact maternel et néonatal des Recommandations pour la pratique clinique du CNGOF relatives à l'épisiotomie. Étude unicentrique à propos de 5409 accouchements par voie vaginale. Gynécologie Obs Fertil. 2009;37(9):697-702. DOI:10.1016/J.GYOBFE.2009.06.003

[17] Ma K, Byrd L. Episiotomy: What angle do you cut to the midline? Eur J Obstet Gynecol Reprod Biol. 2017;213:102-106. DOI:10.1016/j.ejogrb.2017.04.006

[18] Reynolds JL. Reducing the frequency of episiotomies through a continuous quality improvement program. CMAJ. 1995;153(3):275-282. http://www.ncbi.nlm.nih.gov/pubmed/7614443. Accessed December 12, 2019.

[19] Steiner N, Weintraub AY, Wiznitzer A, Sergienko R, Sheiner E. Episiotomy: The final cut? Arch Gynecol Obstet. 2012;286(6):1369-1373. DOI:10.1007/s00404-012-2460-x

[20] Sheiner E, Levy A, Walfisch A, Hallak M, Mazor M. Third degree perineal tears in a university medical center where midline episiotomies are not performed. Arch Gynecol Obstet. 2005;271(4):307-310. DOI:10.1007/s00404-004-0610-5

[21] Carroli G, Mignini L. Episiotomy for vaginal birth. Cochrane database Syst Rev. 2009;(1):CD000081. DOI:10.1002/14651858.CD000081.pub2

[22] Vendittelli F, Rivière O, Crenn-Hébert C, et al. Réseau Sentinelle Audipog 2004-2005. Partie 2: évaluation des pratiques professionnelles. Gynécologie Obs Fertil. 2008;36(12): 1202-1210. DOI:10.1016/J.GYOBFE.2008.08.011

[23] Frass KA, Al-Harazi AH. Episiotomy is still performed routinely in Yemeni women. Saudi Med J. 2010;31(7):764-767. http://www.ncbi.nlm.nih.gov/pubmed/20635009. Accessed January 6, 2020.

[24] Räisänen S, Selander T, Cartwright R, et al. The Association of Episiotomy with Obstetric Anal Sphincter Injury – A Population Based Matched Cohort Study. Obukhov AG, ed. PLoS One. 2014;9(9):e107053. DOI:10.1371/journal.pone.0107053

[25] Räisänen S, Cartwright R, Gissler M, et al. Changing associations of episiotomy and anal sphincter injury across risk strata: Results of a population-based register study in Finland 2004-2011. BMJ Open. 2013;3(8):e003216. DOI:10.1136/bmjopen-2013-003216

[26] Andrews V, Sultan AH, Thakar R, Jones PW. Occult anal sphincter injuries – Myth or reality? BJOG An Int J Obstet Gynaecol. 2006. DOI:10.1111/j.1471-0528.2006.00799.x

[27] Bick DE, Ismail KM, Macdonald S, Thomas P, Tohill S, Kettle C. How good are we at implementing evidence to support the management of birth related perineal trauma? A UK wide survey of midwifery practice. BMC Pregnancy Childbirth. 2012;12. DOI:10.1186/1471-2393-12-57

[28] Cornet A, Porta O, Piñeiro L, Ferriols E, Gich I, Calaf J. Management of Obstetric Perineal Tears: Do obstetrics and gynaecology residents receive adequate training? Results of an anonymous survey. Obstet Gynecol Int. 2012. DOI:10.1155/2012/316983

[29] Wong KW, Ravindran K, Thomas JM, Andrews V. Mediolateral episiotomy: Are trained midwives and doctors approaching it from a different angle? Eur J Obstet Gynecol Reprod Biol. 2014;174:46-50. DOI:10.1016/j.ejogrb.2013.12.002

[30] Gonzalez-Díaz E, Fernández Fernández C, Fernández Corona A. Differences in characteristics of mediolateral episiotomy in proffesionals at the same hospital. J Matern Neonatal Med. September 2015:1-5. DOI:10.3109/14767058.2015.1086328

Section 2

Clinical Management of Pelvic Floor Disorders

Chapter 4

Therapeutic Effect of Magnetic Stimulation Therapy on Pelvic Floor Muscle Dysfunction

Takuro Kobayashi, Toshiyuki China, Naoko Takazawa, Fumitaka Shimizu, Julius Fink, Shigeo Horie and Tomohiro Imai

Abstract

Pelvic bottom dysfunction includes sexual dysfunction, lower urinary tract dysfunction, defecation dysfunction, etc., and the quality of daily life is significantly impaired. Although drug based and surgical therapies exist as treatment methods, non-invasive treatment methods for pelvic floor dysfunction are highly desired, and magnetic stimulation therapy is attracting attention as a potential new approach. Magnetic stimulation therapy can generate deeper stimulations as compared to electrical stimulation therapy, is less painful, and can be performed while wearing clothes. In addition, it is a very safe treatment method with only few reports of side effects. From nocturnal enuresis in children to middle-aged sexual dysfunction and urinary incontinence in the elderly, therapeutic effects on various pelvic floor dysfunctions have been confirmed regardless of age and gender. It is expected that magnetic therapy will continue to develop as a new therapy in the futures. This chapter first describes the pelvic floor muscles and the principles of anatomy and magnetic therapy. In addition, the therapeutic effects of magnetic therapy will be explained in detail one by one. We will also explain the potential application of magnetic therapy for sarcopenia, which is a problem in our aging society.

Keywords: magnetic stimulation therapy, pelvic floor muscles, urinary incontinence, men's health, sarcopenia

1. Introduction

The pelvis contains organs such as the bladder, prostate, (uterus in women), and rectum, and the pelvic floor muscles are the underlying muscles. The pelvic floor muscles wrap around the pelvic bones and support several organs. Some pelvic floor muscles form a sling around the rectum for greater stability. The functioning of these pelvic floor muscles maintains urination, defecation, and sexual life. However, if the muscles at the bottom of the pelvis cannot be properly relaxed during urination or defecation, urinary incontinence, fecal incontinence, ED, and women will experience pain during sexual intercourse.

Pelvic bottom dysfunction (PFD) is a disease caused by damage, dysfunction, and degeneration of pelvic bottom supporting tissue, which is advocated by the International Urological Society (IUGA) and the International Continence Society (ICS). It mainly includes pelvic organ prolapse (POP), pelvic pain, sexual dysfunction, lower urinary tract (LUT) abnormality, and defecation dysfunction. The causes of such pelvic floor muscle dysfunction are not known at all, but aging, obesity, pregnancy, pelvic surgery, etc. are known as factors.

The first non-invasive treatment proposed for pelvic floor muscle dysfunction is pelvic floor muscle training (PFMT), but the results are inconsistent. Systematic review and meta-analysis of non-surgical treatments for urinary incontinence, examining combinations of five common interventions: PFMT, electrical stimulation (ES), vaginal cone (VC), bladder training (BT), and serotonin-noradrenaline reuptake inhibitors (SNRIs). This study reported that more intense PFMT was an effective treatment, but incontinence assessment methods and intervention protocols differed between studies, and further research is needed [1]. Given the difficulty and effectiveness of sustaining PFMT, new conservative therapies are needed to replace pelvic floor muscle training.

In recent years, the US Food and Drug Administration has approved magnetic stimulation as a new non-invasive treatment method for pelvic floor muscle dysfunction. Magnetic stimulation therapy is a method of non-invasively stimulating central nerves and peripheral nerves using electric current generated by magnetism. This method was previously used in the fields of neurology and orthopedics as transcranial magnetic stimulation and skeletal muscle magnetic stimulation, but in the field of urology, it is mainly used for the treatment of urinary incontinence. Furthermore, magnetic stimulation therapy has been found to be effective not only in urinary incontinence but also in a series of diseases related to the pelvic floor muscles.

This paper focuses on magnetic stimulation therapy and introduces various therapeutic effects on pelvic floor muscle disorders.

2. Functional anatomy of the pelvic floor muscles

The bottom of the pelvis has a three-layer structure from the upper part to the visceral pelvic diaphragm, the pelvic diaphragm, and the urogenital diaphragm. The target approach to the pelvic floor muscles is the muscles in the second layer of the pelvic diaphragm. The pelvic diaphragm mainly consists of the levator ani and coccygeus muscles. The levator ani muscle consists of medial and lateral muscles, and the medial pubococcygeus is inside the levator ani tendon arch, originating from the pelvic fascial tendon arch, supporting the outside of the vagina and rectum, and attaches to the anterior sacrococcygeal ligament. The lateral iliococccygeus muscle begins at the levator ani tendon arch and attaches to the tip and lateral edge of the coccyx. The levator ani and coccygeus muscles form the pelvic diaphragm and close the pelvic outlet. The left and right levator ani muscles do not intersect in the center and form a fissure that penetrates the urethra, vagina, and rectum. On the other hand, the coccygeus muscle covers the inner surface of the ischial spine to the inner surface of the sacral ligament and attaches to the lower part of the sacrum and the outer edge of the coccyx.

3. Motor function of the pelvic floor muscles

The pelvic floor muscles support the organs and are active at rest. Therefore, the pelvic floor muscle group is composed of slow muscle fibers that act as posture maintenance at a high rate. Furthermore, the pelvic floor muscles do not work alone, and when the pelvic floor muscles are contracted, the abdominal muscles contract, and conversely, when the abdominal muscles are contracted, the pelvic floor muscles are also activated. When the abdominal pressure rises, the pelvic floor muscles and abdominal muscles move inward. However, in cases of dysfunction of the pelvic floor muscle group such as urinary incontinence, the pelvic floor muscle group and the abdominal muscle move outward [2].

4. What is magnetic stimulation therapy?

4.1 Principle of magnetic stimulation therapy

When an electric current is passed through the coil, a magnetic field is generated along the coil axis. An electric field is induced in proportion to the rate of change of the magnetic field, stimulating skeletal muscle, the autonomic nervous system, and the somatic nervous system. When a pulsed current is passed through the coil of a chair, a pulsed magnetic field is generated in the pelvis and an eddy current is generated. The eddy current stimulates the pelvic floor muscles, which are mainly the pelvic nerve, and suppresses the pelvic nerve and stimulates the lower abdominal nerve via the afferent fibers of the pelvic nerve and bladder, and the urinary muscle. As a result, the pressure in the urethra increases and bladder contraction is suppressed.

4.2 Advantages and disadvantages of magnetic stimulation therapy

There are three major advantages of magnetic stimulation therapy compared to electrical stimulation therapy. One is the depth of stimulation. Magnetic stimulation therapy can stimulate nerves deeper than electrical stimulation. Currently, in Japan, a chair-type stimulator that magnetically stimulates the area around the anus is used. Such stimulation of deep nerves is difficult to reproduce with electrical stimulation therapy.

The second is that it can be done non-invasively. Since the magnetic stimulation penetrates clothes, skin, bones, etc., it can be performed while wearing clothes without inserting an anus or vaginal electrodes. Therefore, this treatment method is more comfortable and less embarrassing. Furthermore, the targets to be stimulated are the sacral nerve and the pelvic floor, but treatment can be performed without pain often observed in electrical stimulation.

The third is safety. Magnetic stimulation therapy is considered to be an extremely safe and side-effect-free treatment. In a multicenter, randomized, sham-controlled trial, magnetic stimulation therapy did not show any adverse events compared to the placebo group [3]. This data suggests that magnetic stimulation is safer than electrical stimulation associated with side effects such as abdominal pain and diarrhea [4].

However, there are two major disadvantages. One is the need to go to the hospital. Magnetic therapy does not end with just one treatment, and requires about 8–16 visits in 1 to 2 months. Depending on access to the hospital and the patient's health condition, this might be challenging. The second disadvantage is that this can be a difficult intervention in certain patients. For example, in patients with a pacemaker,

Pros	Cons
• stimulation of nerves in deep muscles • no requirement for dressing change • minimal side effects	• difficult to perform on patients who is with tattoo or a pacemaker.

Table 1.
Pros and cons of magnetic stimulation therapy.

magnetic therapy can cause malfunctions, and in patients with tattoos, the likelihood of burns increases (**Table 1**).

5. Therapeutic effect of magnetic therapy

5.1 Effect on urinary incontinence

Urinary incontinence (UI) is a common urinary disease and is usually defined as involuntary urine leakage due to weakening of the urethral sphincter and pelvic floor muscles without the need for urination [5]. According to the International Continence Association (ICS), urinary incontinence affects more than 200 million people worldwide, primarily women. Half of women may not report UI, perhaps because of embarrassment, lack of knowledge about treatments, and the belief that UI is normal with age. Urinary incontinence can be divided into (i) stress incontinence (ii) urge incontinence (iii) mixed incontinence, which is a combination of the two types. Stress urinary incontinence accounts for 29–75% of women, urge incontinence accounts for 7–33% of the population, and mixed urinary incontinence accounts for 14–61% of the population. Men may also develop urinary incontinence due to urethral sphincter deficiency after radical prostatectomy, adversely affecting the patient's quality of life [6]. Controlling urinary incontinence is also an important issue for extending healthy life expectancy. It is known that the prevalence of urinary incontinence increases with age in the elderly. A large database analysis in Northern California found that the risk of admission to a long-term care facility after diagnosis of urinary incontinence was twice as high for women and 3.2 times for men, and increased the risk of hospitalization [7].

Various research reports have been published on the therapeutic effect of magnetic stimulation on stress urinary incontinence (SUI). In a randomized, double-blind, sham controlled trial of 120 female patients with SUI, the treatment group received magnetic stimulation twice a week for a total of 16 times over a two-month period. When the primary endpoint is a decrease in the score of ICIQ-UI SF (International Consultation on Incontinence Questionnaire for Urinary Incontinence-Short Form) by 5 points as the therapeutic response, the therapeutic response in the magnetic therapy group is 3.46 times that in the placebo group. The total score of ICIQ-UI SF decreased significantly. There was also a consistent significant improvement in score between 1 and 2 months, indicating that 8-week PMS was more effective than 4-week. An additional year of follow-up suggested that the effect was long-lasting [8]. In a pilot study comparing 52 randomized patients with SUI, the treatment group showed lower myostatin levels and improved UI severity ratings (The Revised Urinary Incontinence Scale) and depression severity (Beck Depression Inventory) before and after treatment [9]. In a randomized, sham-controlled trial of 30 female SUI patients resistant to pelvic floor muscle training, magnetic stimulation significantly improved ICIQ-SF and the abdominal leak point pressure (ALPP) in the treatment group compared to baseline, with significant differences between groups ($P < 0.05$). In addition, self-efficacy beliefs (GSES) improved in the magnetic therapy group, and the authors reported that there were effects of magnetic therapy on both physical and psychosocial aspects [10]. In a randomized controlled trial of three groups of women with SUI: a pelvic floor muscle training and extracorporeal magnetic therapy group and a control group, the two treatment groups showed a decrease in depressive symptoms (BDI-II) and significant improvements in an improvement in urinary incontinence severity (RUIS) and several quality of life items (KHQ). Moreover, GSES improved in the extracorporeal magnetic therapy group [11]. A study was also conducted to evaluate the effect of sacral magnetic stimulation (SMS) on functional and urodynamic improvement in patients 45–75 years of age with refractory SUI. This study was a sham-controlled, double-blind, parallel study with a follow-up of 4.5 months [12]. Compared to the sham group, the experimental group showed significant improvement in Urge-Urinary Distress Inventory and Overactive Bladder Questionnaire (OAB-q) scores after the intervention and also at follow-up. In addition, there were significant increases in bladder capacity, urethral functional length, and pressure transmission ratio after the intervention. The response to SMS was greater in patients with severe SUI than in patients with mild symptoms, confirming the effectiveness of SMS in the treatment of SUI. In another study, a total of 75 patients with stress urinary incontinence were subjected to repetitive magnetic stimulation of 15 Hz. at the sacral root at 50% intensity output for 30 minutes with a duration of 5 seconds per minute. As a result, an obvious increase in urethral closing pressure and a significant increase in bladder capacity after stimulation were observed in the sacral stimulation group. In addition, the number of urine leaks and urine volume in the pad test were significantly decreased in the active stimulation group than in the sham stimulation group, and the QOL score was also significantly improved. The improvement rate of the active stimulation group was 74%, which was significantly higher than that of the sham stimulation group (32%) [13]. A randomized controlled trial investigating the short- and long-term effects of repetitive magnetic stimulation on the sacral root observed an improvement in the quality of life of patients with abdominal stress urinary incontinence at one week after stimulation [14].

Some studies have reported therapeutic effects on urge and mixed urinary incontinence. In a multicenter, randomized, single-blind, controlled trial of 151 women with urge incontinence with overactive bladder, armchair-type magnetic stimulators were used to stimulate magnetically twice a week for 25 minutes. As a result, the number of urine leaks / week according to the bladder diary was significantly improved in the treatment group, and the urgency within 24 hours and the average excretion amount were also significantly improved. In addition, the change in total OABSS from baseline was significantly lower in the treatment group than in the sham group, and the change in mean IPSS-QOL score was also significantly lower in the treatment group [3]. A retrospective study conducted in Italy examined the effects of magnetic therapy on 20 men and women with stress incontinence, urge incontinence, and mixed incontinence. The treatment was performed using a functional magnetic stimulator and a magnetic coil installed under the seating surface of the chair. During treatment, the patient was instructed to sit in a chair so that the perineum was centered on the coil and that muscle contractions (pelvic floor and sphincter contractions) were felt during stimulation. Patients were treated for 20 minutes / session, twice a week for 3 weeks (6 times in total). The stimulation frequency was fixed at 10 Hz for 10 minutes and at 35 Hz for another 10 minutes, and the activity time and rest time were 6 seconds each. As a result, micturition frequency and nocturia were significantly reduced before and after treatment, and bladder capacity was significantly increased [15]. A study of 82 female patients with various urinary incontinences in Slovenia received 10 magnetic stimuli over a 4-week period. As a result, in urge incontinence and mixed incontinence, the frequency of urinary incontinence, the number of daily urinary incontinence, and the decrease in the number of urination were statistically observed [16].

5.1.1 Postoperative urinary incontinence of prostate cancer

Prostate cancer is the number one cancer in Europe and the United States that affects men. Surgery and radiation therapy are used for localized prostate cancer. Although surgical invasion has been significantly reduced due to the spread of surgical robot Da Vinci technique in recent years, postoperative stress urinary incontinence caused by removal of the prostate reduces the patient's QOL. In a multicenter study in the United States, 46% of patients required a urinary incontinence pad 6 months after surgery, and urinary incontinence often persists long after surgery [17]. In a previous study, 10 patients who had been suffering from urinary incontinence for more than 12 months after radical prostatectomy were treated with magnetic therapy for 20 minutes, twice a week for 2 months. The pulsed field frequency was 10 Hz for 10 minutes, followed by a second treatment at 50 Hz for 10 minutes. As objective and subjective evaluations, a micturition diary, a 1-hour pad weight test, and a quality of life survey were performed 1, 2, 3, and 6 months after the start of treatment. As a result, 30% of patients became dry and 30% showed improvement. In the 1-hour pad weight test, the average pad weight decreased from 25 to 10.3 g, and the QOL score improved significantly 2 months after treatment. In addition, the number of urine leaks per day decreased from 5.0 before treatment to 1.9 after treatment [18]. Although robotic surgery has improved the degree of urinary incontinence, 14% of patients in our department still use two or more urinary incontinence pads/day after 6 months post surgery. In order to improve this annoying complication after surgery, our facility is currently actively adopting magnetic therapy.

5.2 Effect on detrusor overactivity

Detrusor overactivity is a common cause of urge incontinence in elderly and young patients. It occurs when the detrusor muscle contracts intermittently for no apparent reason when the bladder is partially or almost completely filled. Detrusor overactivity can be idiopathic or due to dysfunction of the detrusor center of the frontal lobe (generally due to age-related changes, dementia, or stroke) or lower urinary tract obstruction. Urinary muscle overactivity with contractile force disorder is a variant of urgency urinary incontinence, characterized by urinary urgency, pollakiuria, decreased urinary retention, urinary retention, bladder pillar formation, and post-micturition residual urine volume of over 50 mL. In a study comparing magnetic therapy with the placebo group for idiopathic detrusor hyperactivity, the magnetic therapy group significantly reduced the number of micturitions per day compared to the placebo group. It was also confirmed that the number of urination and QOL per day improved although the sample size was not sufficient [19].

In a randomized controlled trial of 32 men and women comparing the effects of magnetic and electrical stimulation, a significant increase in bladder capacity was found in the magnetic stimulation group [20].

5.3 Effect on neurogenic overactive bladder

Neurogenic bladder is a lower urinary tract dysfunction caused by a neurological disorder, and the diagnosis is based on urodynamic testing. When the upper part of the pontine detrusor center existing in the brain stem is damaged, neurogenic detrusor overactivity causes the bladder to contract involuntarily against the intention of the person occurs, resulting in urge incontinence and pollakiuria. In a study comparing the effects of pulsed electromagnetic field therapy (PEMFT) and transcutaneous electrical nerve stimulation (TENS) on neuropathic overactive bladder dysfunction in patients with spinal cord injury (SCI), 50 male and 30 female patients (average age of 40 years) with secondary neuropathic overactive bladder due to spinal cord injury were recruited. Urinary tract dynamics (UDS) were performed before and after treatment. 40 patients received TENS (10 Hz, 700 second pulse) 3 times/week, for a total of 20 times and the remaining 40 patients received PEMFT (15 Hz, 50% intensity 5) 3 times/week, for a total of 20 times. As a result, the maximum cystometric capacity, volume at first uninhibited detrusor contraction, and maximum urinary flow rate were significantly increased in the PEMFT group, indicating that PEMFT is superior to TENS in terms of therapeutic effect [21].

5.4 Effect on bedwetting

Nocturnal enuresis is usually the involuntary urination during sleep after the age at which bladder control begins. According to the American Psychiatric Association's DSM-IV, primary nocturnal enuresis (PNE) was described as "children 5 years and older who repeatedly urinate in bed and clothing twice a week for at least 3 consecutive months, not resulting from side effects and medical conditions of drugs. " Nocturnal urine in children and adults causes mental stress and sometimes causes complications such as urinary tract infections. A study evaluating the potential clinical and urodynamic effects of functional magnetic stimulation (FMS) in the treatment of girls with primary nocturnal enuresis (PNE) compared to placebo reported the effects of magnetic therapy. 20 PNE girls (average age of 10.8 years) were given a magnetic stimulator for 2 months day and night, the number of episodes of nocturnal urine decreased from 3.1 to 1.3 times a week in the magnetic therapy group before and after treatment. In addition, the bladder volume at the strong desire to void increased significantly compared with the placebo group [22].

Monosymptomatic nocturnal enuresis (MNE) refers to patients with nocturnal enuresis without other lower urinary tract symptoms such as daytime urinary incontinence and urgency. In a study that randomly assigned 44 patients with MNE to receive 10 sets of repetitive sacral root magnetic stimulation (rSMS), the treatment group significantly improved the mean nocturnal urine per week compared to the placebo group. The effect was maintained even 1 month after the treatment. The treatment group also showed improvement in visual analog scale (VAS) and quality of life [23].

5.5 Effect on chronic pelvic pain syndrome

Chronic pelvic pain syndrome includes inflammation of the prostate gland, pain from the lower abdomen to the lower body, discomfort around the pelvic body, urinary symptoms such as close urine and feeling of residual urine, discomfort during ejaculation, and erectile dysfunction. It is a disease reminding of sexual dysfunction. Although the exact causes have not been clarified yet, blood flow disorders and autoimmune reactions around the prostate gland, urine reflux into the prostate gland due to dysuria, sensory nerve abnormalities in the pelvis and lower body, adrenal gland hormones and abnormalities in sex hormones are believed to be the causes. It is often seen in relatively young people (late teens to 40s), and the symptoms worsen when the perineal area is compressed by a long sitting posture (desk work, driving a car, bicycle, motorcycle, etc.).

In addition, psychological stress, fatigue, smoking, excessive drinking, and poor circulation are also factors that worsen the symptoms. It is characterized by the absence of typical symptoms but various symptoms from the lower abdomen to the lower body start to appear. Pain may be felt not only in the perineum near the prostate, but also in areas not related to the prostate, such as the lower back, urethra, groin, thighs, and lower abdomen. In addition, it may be accompanied by urinary symptoms such as close urine, feeling of residual urine, weak urine momentum, pain in the urethra when urinating, and sexual dysfunction such as discomfort during ejaculation and erectile disorder.

A randomized, placebo-controlled, double-blind study of 60 men with refractory chronic pelvic pain syndrome evaluated improvement in the Chronic Prostatic Inflammatory Symptom Index (NIH-CPSI) of the National Institutes of Health. The QOL score was significantly improved 12 weeks after treatment compared to the placebo group. In addition, patients with persistent symptoms of 1 year or less were more effective than patients with long-lasting symptoms [24].

On the other hand, there are also studies in which randomized, double-blind, placebo-controlled treatment was used for chronic pelvic pain in women. In this study, 32 patients with chronic pelvic pain were treated with active magnets (500G) or placebo magnets 24 hours a day at trigger points in the abdomen. After 1 month of treatment, McGill Pain Questionnaire, Pain Disability Index and Clinical Global Impressions Scale were evaluated. As a result, the Pain Disability Index, Clinical Global Impressions-Severity, and Clinical Global Impressions-Improvement were significantly lower in the treatment group than in the placebo group, demonstrating the therapeutic effect of magnetic therapy [25].

5.6 Effect on fecal incontinence

Fecal incontinence is defined as an involuntary leak of liquid or solid stool that poses a social or hygienic problem. Fecal incontinence is not life-threatening, but it is an intolerable symptom for patients and significantly impairs their quality of life. The prevalence of fecal incontinence over the age of 65 in Japan is 8.7% for men and 6.6% for women. In the elderly, the onset of fecal incontinence often triggers admission to a facility, and it is thought that even for home care recipients, the most worrying thing about caregivers is receiving excretory care. Fecal incontinence is classified into leaky fecal incontinence, in which stool leaks without being noticed, urgent fecal incontinence, in which stool leaks without being able to endure the toilet, and mixed fecal incontinence, which is a mixture of both. It is roughly divided into. Leaky fecal incontinence is more likely to occur when the internal anal sphincter is impaired, and urgent fecal incontinence is more likely to occur when the external anal sphincter is impaired. The internal anal sphincter muscles often weaken with age, and the external anal sphincter muscles are often injured by labor or surgery for rectal cancer.

Surgical treatments for fecal incontinence include sacral stimulation therapy, anal sphincter plasty, and stoma construction. From the viewpoint of evidence and invasiveness, it is desirable to try non-invasive therapies first. Non-invasive therapies include diet / lifestyle / defecation habit guidance, drug therapy, pelvic floor muscle training, biofeedback therapy, butt plugs, and retrograde intestinal lavage (irrigation defecation). The objectives are fecal solidification, increased contractility of the pelvic floor muscles, including the external anal sphincter, normalization of rectal sensation, and regular emptiness of the rectum and colon.

In a study reporting the effects of magnetic therapy on fecal incontinence, 10 patients with fecal incontinence with an average age of 57 years received perineal magnetic stimulation (10 Hz and 50 Hz) twice weekly for 5 weeks. Both 10 Hz and 50 Hz stimulation significantly increased anal pressure compared to baseline rest. After treatment, anal pressure increased significantly and the score for fecal incontinence improved significantly [26].

6. Application to men's health

Erectile dysfunction (ED), one of the male sexual dysfunctions, is defined as persistent or recurrent erections that are insufficient or unsustainable for satisfactory sexual activity. ED is the second most common sexual problem in men after premature ejaculation, and epidemiological studies indicate that it affects 30 million people in the United States. ED has a strong negative impact on self-esteem and self-confidence, can reduce the quality of life for men and their partners, and can affect all aspects of life. The pathophysiology of ED includes angiogenic, neurogenic, anatomical, hormonal, drug-induced, and / or psychogenic causes.

Risk factors for ED include aging, diabetes, obesity and lack of exercise, cardiovascular disease and hypertension, smoking, chronic kidney disease, lower urinary tract symptoms, neurological disorders, depressive symptoms, drugs, sleep apnea syndrome, etc. As a treatment, oral preparations such as sildenafil and intraspinal injection are used. However, patients often change treatment methods due to lack of therapeutic effects and the high costs. Therefore, a therapeutic approach that emphasizes long-term satisfaction is needed.

The magnetic field induces an alternating current in the electrolyte in the body, which affects the water content of cells, mitochondrial function, nutrition, oxygen, amino acid uptake, energy production, etc. Appropriate magnetic fields can increase the uptake of oxygen by cells, promote blood circulation, and restore dysfunction. In a canine study, magnetic stimulation of the corpus cavernosum nerve increased intracavitary pressure, resulting in a complete penis erection after an incubation period of approximately 8 seconds. Upon discontinuation of stimulation, erection and intracavitary pressure returned to baseline after an average of 14 seconds [27]. In a study of 32 neuropathic ED patients and 20 healthy volunteers, a magnetic coil was placed on the dorsal side of the penis near the symphysis pubis, with 40% strength, 20 Hz frequency, and 50 seconds of magnetism. The stimulation was performed, and 50 seconds later, the magnetic stimulation was stopped. As a result, the magnetic therapy group was able to induce penile stiffness non-invasively without side effects [28]. A double-blind, placebo-controlled trial evaluating the effectiveness of impulse magnetic-field therapy for psychogenic erectile dysfunction or orgasmic disorders has also been reported [29]. Twenty men between the ages of 30 and 60 who suffered from ED and orgasm dysfunction were treated with Impulse magnetic-field therapy for 3 weeks, and the treatment group showed improved erection intensity, duration, well-being and sexual activity as compared to the placebo group [29]. No side effects from treatment were reported.

The data above supports the effectiveness of magnetic therapy for various types of ED, drawing more and more attention to magnetic therapy in the men's health community.

7. Frail and sarcopenia

Frail is a state that shows vulnerability to external stress with aging, and is said to be different from the state requiring nursing care. There is no global definition of frailty or diagnostic criteria, but Fried's criteria are widely adopted [30]. It has been pointed out that the onset of frailty is related to the decrease in hormone levels such as sex hormones and vitamin D, nutritional status and nutrient intake, and the relationship between low testosterone status and frailty syndrome, physical function, and fall risk [31]. In addition, a study analyzing the relationship between frailty and urinary incontinence in 300 elderly people in Italy found that elderly people with urinary incontinence were at significantly higher risk of being classified as frailty, and urinary incontinence is a marker of frailty in the elderly [32].

Sarcopenia's pathology is similar to the frailty syndrome and is also a major contributor to the physical frailty syndrome, defined as age-related loss of muscle mass and strength. Frail's phenotype can be broadly divided into five types. That is, malnutrition (weight loss), subjective decreased vitality (easy fatigue), decreased activity, decreased mobility (decreased walking speed), and decreased muscle strength (decreased grip strength). Of these, weakness and weakness are called physical frailty and are elements of sarcopenia. Sarcopenia has been attracting attention in recent years as a cause of bedridden and fall risk in the elderly. The prevalence of sarcopenia is estimated to be approximately 9% in young women and approximately 18% in older men [33]. The causes of sarcopenia are qualitative changes accompanied by functional decline such as fast muscle fiber-specific atrophy, decreased fiber count, and connective tissue hyperplasia due to changes in nutritional status, decreased physical activity, and production of inflammatory cytokines.

Eddy currents caused by magnetic stimulation induce contraction of skeletal muscle by causing depolarization of cell membranes of peripheral nerves and skeletal muscle. Electrical stimulation has been widely used in the clinical setting of conventional rehabilitation, but rehabilitation by painless magnetic stimulation is expected in the future. In addition, a study examining the relationship between sarcopenia and ADL in patients with early-stage Alzheimer's suggests that disorientation and sarcopenia may interact to induce functional urinary incontinence. In addition, another study examining the correlation between dysuria and the overall functioning of the elderly found a significant correlation between urinary storage symptoms and the Barthel Index, suggesting that improvement in dysuria leads to improvement in symptoms, including sarcopenia. From these reports, magnetic therapy is expected to improve muscle mass and dysuria in sarcopenia patients, and may be a breakthrough non-invasive therapy in our aging society.

8. Current status of magnetic therapy in Japan and our efforts

In Japan, insurance is applied to female patients with intractable overactive bladder who do not improve their symptoms even after taking a urinary incontinence drug

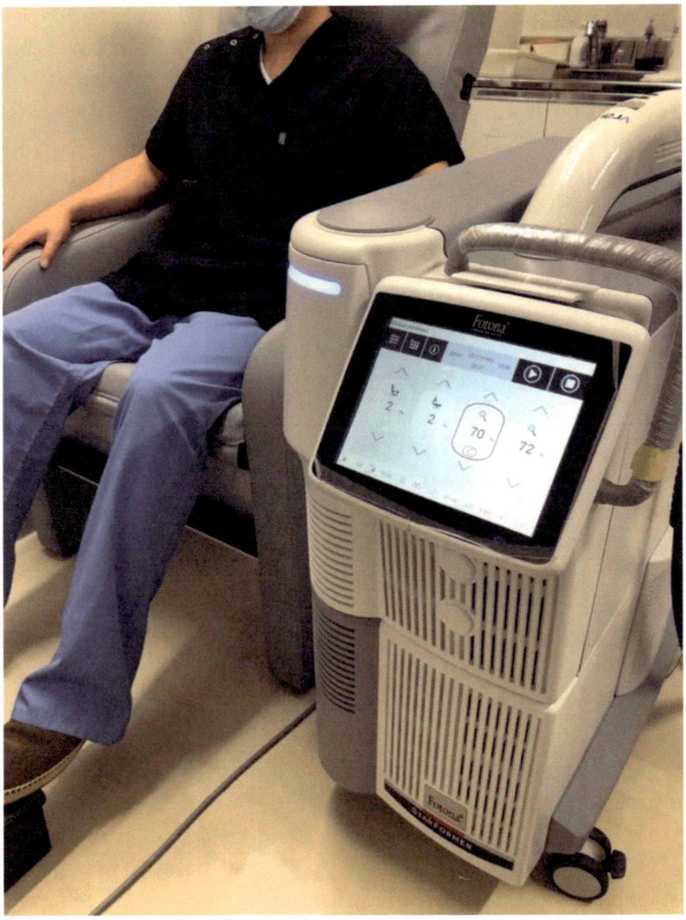

Figure 1.
A device of magnetic stimulation therapy (Starformer by Fotona).

for 12 weeks or more, or who cannot use the drug due to the side effects of the drug. Insurance can be calculated up to 2 courses per year, with 6 weeks as 1 course, up to 25 minutes each time, up to 2 times a week. Considering reports from other countries, the usefulness of magnetic therapy is considered to span multiple diseases, and the therapeutic indication in Japan is still narrow. Therefore, our related facilities are providing treatment to patients with a wide range of diseases by introducing overseas magnetic stimulators (**Figure 1**). Although the number of cases is still small, magnetic therapy is performed for 20 to 30 minutes at a time, 1 to 2 times a week, for a total of 8 times as one course. Comparing the questionnaires before and after the treatment, both men and women showed improvement in nocturia, urinary incontinence, and sexual dysfunction in men, and felt the effectiveness of magnetic treatment. In fact, patients said "the number of nighttime urinations did not improve with drug therapy or physical therapy but decreased from 3 to 1 since I started magnetic therapy", "the intervals between urination has increased and it has become easier during the day and night", "urine leakage has improved and pad replacement has decreased", "erectile power has improved", and "I have improved my back pain after magnetic therapy." If the effect is poor in one cool, a second cool is recommended, and might improve the effects. I feel that it is necessary to increase the number of cases in future in order to expand the scope of application of magnetic therapy in Japan.

9. Conclusions

Magnetic therapy is a safe, non-invasive treatment that could be potentially used to treat pollakiuria, incontinence, men's health, and sarcopenia. With further research evidence in the future, it may become the gold standard for the initial treatment of pelvic dysfunction.

Acknowledgements

The authors appreciate the technical support of Tokyo Kekkan-Geka Clinic, Tokyo, Japan.

Conflict of interest

The authors have no conflict of interest.

Author details

Takuro Kobayashi[1], Toshiyuki China[1], Naoko Takazawa[1], Fumitaka Shimizu[1], Julius Fink[1], Shigeo Horie[1*] and Tomohiro Imai[2]

1 Department of Urology, Juntendo University Graduate School of Medicine, Tokyo, Japan

2 Tokyo Kekkan-Geka Clinic, Tokyo, Japan

*Address all correspondence to: shorie@juntendo.ac.jp

References

[1] Imamura M, Abrams P, Bain C, Buckley B, Cardozo L, Cody J, et al. Systematic review and economic modelling of the effectiveness and cost-effectiveness of non-surgical treatments for women with stress urinary incontinence. Health Technol Assess. 2010;14:1-188, iii-iv.

[2] Sapsford R. Rehabilitation of pelvic floor muscles utilizing trunk stabilization. Man Ther. 2004;9:3-12.

[3] Yamanishi T, Homma Y, Nishizawa O, Yasuda K, Yokoyama O, Group S-XS. Multicenter, randomized, sham-controlled study on the efficacy of magnetic stimulation for women with urgency urinary incontinence. Int J Urol. 2014;21:395-400.

[4] Schreiner L, Santos TG, Souza AB, Nygaard CC, Silva Filho IG. Electrical stimulation for urinary incontinence in women: a systematic review. Int Braz J Urol. 2013;39:454-464.

[5] Lin CS, Lue TF. Stem cell therapy for stress urinary incontinence: a critical review. Stem Cells Dev. 2012;21:834-843.

[6] Radadia KD, Farber NJ, Shinder B, Polotti CF, Milas LJ, Tunuguntla H. Management of Postradical Prostatectomy Urinary Incontinence: A Review. Urology. 2018;113:13-19.

[7] Thom DH, Haan MN, Van Den Eeden SK. Medically recognized urinary incontinence and risks of hospitalization, nursing home admission and mortality. Age Ageing. 1997;26:367-374.

[8] Lim R, Liong ML, Leong WS, Karim Khan NA, Yuen KH. Pulsed Magnetic Stimulation for Stress Urinary Incontinence: 1-Year Followup Results. J Urol. 2017;197:1302-1308.

[9] Weber-Rajek M, Radziminska A, Straczynska A, Podhorecka M, Kozakiewicz M, Perkowski R, et al. A randomized-controlled trial pilot study examining the effect of extracorporeal magnetic innervation in the treatment of stress urinary incontinence in women. Clin Interv Aging. 2018;13:2473-2480.

[10] Yamanishi T, Suzuki T, Sato R, Kaga K, Kaga M, Fuse M. Effects of magnetic stimulation on urodynamic stress incontinence refractory to pelvic floor muscle training in a randomized sham-controlled study. Low Urin Tract Symptoms. 2019;11:61-65.

[11] Weber-Rajek M, Straczynska A, Strojek K, Piekorz Z, Pilarska B, Podhorecka M, et al. Assessment of the Effectiveness of Pelvic Floor Muscle Training (PFMT) and Extracorporeal Magnetic Innervation (ExMI) in Treatment of Stress Urinary Incontinence in Women: A Randomized Controlled Trial. Biomed Res Int. 2020;2020:1019872.

[12] Tsai PY, Wang CP, Hsieh CY, Tsai YA, Yeh SC, Chuang TY. Long-term sacral magnetic stimulation for refractory stress urinary incontinence. Arch Phys Med Rehabil. 2014;95:2231-2238.

[13] Fujishiro T, Enomoto H, Ugawa Y, Takahashi S, Ueno S, Kitamura T. Magnetic stimulation of the sacral roots for the treatment of stress incontinence: an investigational study and placebo controlled trial. J Urol. 2000;164:1277-1279.

[14] Manganotti P, Zaina F, Vedovi E, Pistoia L, Rubilotta E, D'Amico A, et al. Repetitive magnetic stimulation of the sacral roots for the treatment of stress incontinence: a brief report. Eura Medicophys. 2007;43:339-344.

[15] Vadala M, Palmieri B, Malagoli A, Laurino C. High-power Magnetotherapy:

A New Weapon in Urinary Incontinence? Low Urin Tract Symptoms. 2018;10: 266-270.

[16] Štrumbelj T, Logar T, Podnar P, Mežek ZK, Zorec B. Stress incontinence and after childbirth incontinence treatment using magneto stym neuromuscular stimulator. Journal of Croatian Society of Physiotherapists. 2016;14:42-45.

[17] Donovan JL, Hamdy FC, Lane JA, Mason M, Metcalfe C, Walsh E, et al. Patient-Reported Outcomes after Monitoring, Surgery, or Radiotherapy for Prostate Cancer. N Engl J Med. 2016;375:1425-1437.

[18] Yokoyama T, Inoue M, Fujita O, Nozaki K, Nose H, Kumon H. Preliminary results of the effect of extracorporeal magnetic stimulation on urinary incontinence after radical prostatectomy: a pilot study. Urol Int. 2005;74:224-228.

[19] Morris AR, O'Sullivan R, Dunkley P, Moore KH. Extracorporeal magnetic stimulation is of limited clinical benefit to women with idiopathic detrusor overactivity: a randomized sham controlled trial. Eur Urol. 2007;52:876-881.

[20] Yamanishi T, Sakakibara R, Uchiyama T, Suda S, Hattori T, Ito H, et al. Comparative study of the effects of magnetic versus electrical stimulation on inhibition of detrusor overactivity. Urology. 2000;56:777-781.

[21] Fergany LA, Shaker H, Arafa M, Elbadry MS. Does sacral pulsed electromagnetic field therapy have a better effect than transcutaneous electrical nerve stimulation in patients with neurogenic overactive bladder? Arab J Urol. 2017;15:148-152.

[22] But I, Varda NM. Functional magnetic stimulation: a new method for the treatment of girls with primary nocturnal enuresis? J Pediatr Urol. 2006;2:415-418.

[23] Khedr EM, Elbeh KA, Abdel Baky A, Abo-Elfetoh N, El-Hammady DH, Korashy F. A double-blind randomized clinical trial on the efficacy of magnetic sacral root stimulation for the treatment of Monosymptomatic Nocturnal Enuresis. Restor Neurol Neurosci. 2015;33:435-445.

[24] Kessler TM, Mordasini L, Weisstanner C, Juni P, da Costa BR, Wiest R, et al. Sono-electro-magnetic therapy for treating chronic pelvic pain syndrome in men: a randomized, placebo-controlled, double-blind trial. PLoS One. 2014;9:e113368.

[25] Brown CS, Ling FW, Wan JY, Pilla AA. Efficacy of static magnetic field therapy in chronic pelvic pain: a double-blind pilot study. Am J Obstet Gynecol. 2002;187:1581-1587.

[26] Thornton MJ, Kennedy ML, Lubowski DZ. Extracorporeal magnetic stimulation of the pelvic floor: impact on anorectal function and physiology. A pilot study. Dis *Colon Rectum*. 2005;48: 1945-1950.

[27] Shafik A. Penile erection in dogs by magnetic stimulation of the cavernous nerve. Arch Androl. 1999;43:247-252.

[28] Shafik A, el-Sibai O, Shafik AA. Magnetic stimulation of the cavernous nerve for the treatment of erectile dysfunction in humans. Int J Impot Res. 2000;12:137-141; discussion 41-2.

[29] Pelka RB, Jaenicke C, Gruenwald J. Impulse magnetic-field therapy for erectile dysfunction: a double-blind, placebo-controlled study. Adv Ther. 2002;19:53-60.

[30] Fried LP, Tangen CM, Walston J, Newman AB, Hirsch C, Gottdiener J, et al. Frailty in older adults: evidence for

a phenotype. J Gerontol A Biol Sci Med Sci. 2001;56:M146-M156.

[31] Morley JE, Kaiser FE, Sih R, Hajjar R, Perry HM, 3rd. Testosterone and frailty. Clin Geriatr Med. 1997;13: 685-695.

[32] Berardelli M, De Rango F, Morelli M, Corsonello A, Mazzei B, Mari V, et al. Urinary incontinence in the elderly and in the oldest old: correlation with frailty and mortality. Rejuvenation Res. 2013;16:206-211.

[33] Morley JE, Baumgartner RN, Roubenoff R, Mayer J, Nair KS. Sarcopenia. J Lab Clin Med. 2001;137: 231-243.

Chapter 5

Management of Hunner Lesion in Interstitial Cystitis/Bladder Pain Syndrome Patients

Kwang Jin Ko and Kyu-Sung Lee

Abstract

Interstitial cystitis/bladder pain syndrome (IC/BPS) is a chronic condition characterized by chronic pelvic pain related to the bladder. One phenotype of IC/BPS is the Hunner lesion type IC/BPS. Hunner lesion exhibits typical features such as mucosal ulceration, fibrosis, and severe inflammation. The tissue surrounding the Hunner lesion may show lymphoplasmacytic infiltrates, and mast cells are increased in the lamina propria. In this chapter, we discuss intravesical treatment, endoscopic treatment, and partial cystectomy with augmentation cystoplasty for the management of Hunner lesion in IC/BPS patients.

Keywords: Bladder pain syndrome, Endoscopic treatment, Hunner lesion, Interstitial cystitis, Intravesical treatment

1. Introduction

Interstitial cystitis/bladder pain syndrome (IC/BPS) is a condition characterized by chronic pelvic pain, pressure or discomfort perceived to be related to the urinary bladder and is accompanied by other urinary symptoms in the absence of confusable diseases [1]. Interstitial cystitis was first described by Skene in 1887, and its definition has changed over the past 100 years. Guy Hunner was the first to identify the characteristic cytoscopic findings associated with bladder pain that were initially called Hunner's ulcers. However, these cytoscopic findings are not characteristic of an ulcer and instead due to a severe inflammatory lesion; therefore, the term ulcer is no longer used. IC/BPS is divided into the Hunner type interstitial cystitis with Hunner lesion and bladder pain syndrome (BPS) without Hunner lesion [2]. Hunner type IC/BPS cystitis has characteristic endoscopic findings and distinct inflammatory histopathology, whereas BPS lacks both the endoscopic and histopathology findings. The Hunner lesion is described as a "circumscript, reddened mucosal lesion with small vessels radiating toward a central scar, with fibrin deposit or coagulum" and a "velvet red patch that looks like carcinoma in situ" (**Figure 1**) [1].

During cystoscopic examination, it is crucially important to watch the bladder mucosa from the early phase of bladder filling, because Hunner lesions might be obscured shortly after bladder distension. Recent research has revealed significant differences in the demographics, clinical presentation, bladder pathology, urinary marker profiles, and treatment responses between patients with IC/BPS with

IntechOpen

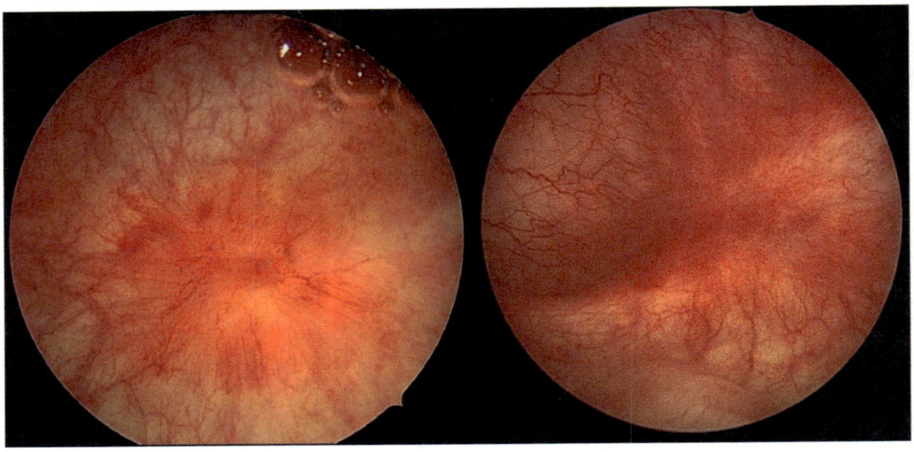

Figure 1.
Cystoscopic findings of Hunner lesion.

Hunner lesion and those without Hunner lesion. IC/BPS with Hunner lesions is a distinct inflammatory disorder characterized by epithelial denudation and frequent clonal expansion of infiltrating B cells, in association with biological processes involved in immune responses and infectious disease [3]. IC/BPS without Hunner lesions, however, rarely show histological changes and retain a preserved urothelium. IC/BPS with Hunner lesion has an incidence of up to 7% among IC/BPS patients and is categorized as a separate disease from non-Hunner IC/BPS [2, 4, 5]. In this chapter, we discuss intravesical treatment and endoscopic treatment of the Hunner lesion type IC/BPS.

2. Intravesical treatment

2.1 Dimethyl sulfoxide

Intravesical instillation of dimethyl sulfoxide (DMSO) was approved by the FDA in 1978 as a treatment method for IC/BPS. The mechanism of action of DMSO may involve anti-inflammatory effects, nerve blockade, smooth muscle relaxation, and collagen inhibition [6]. In the American Urological Association (AUA) guidelines, intravesical DMSO may be used for symptoms refractory to conservative measures or as initial treatment to address severe symptoms as second-line treatment [7]. In contrast, the EAU guideline does not recommend the use of DMSO because of insufficient evidence. A review by Cochrane also reported that the evidence for treating IC/BPS with intravesical DMSO is limited [6]. In 1988, Perez-Marrero et al. [8] published a trial with 33 patients and found that the proportion of patients with subjective symptom improvement was 53% among DMSO-injected patients compared with 18% in the placebo group. Since then, several single-arm studies have been reported, and most studies have confirmed the 61–95% of therapeutic effect of DMSO in patients who did not respond to medication or hydrodistension.

A multicenter, randomized, placebo-controlled trial examining DMSO compared with placebo in 96 patients was recently published in Japan in 2021 [9]. The mean O'Leary-Sant Interstitial Cystitis Symptom Index (ICSI) score at week 12 decreased by −5.2 in the DMSO group compared with a decrease by −3.4 in the placebo group, with a statistically significant difference between the groups. Although the O'Leary-Sant Interstitial Cystitis Problem Index (ICPI), number of frequency, mean voided volume, and maximum voided volume showed significant improvement in the DMSO group compared with placebo group, there was no significant difference in the pain score between the two groups at 12 weeks. In this study, Hunner lesions were confirmed by cystoscopy at baseline in 86% of all patients. The authors speculated that the high incidence of Hunner lesions may have contributed to the clinical efficacy of DMSO. Although it was a small study, another study compared the efficacy of DMSO treatment between patients with and without Hunner lesion, and DMSO intravesical instillation showed a significant therapeutic effect only in IC/BPS patients with Hunner lesion. These findings suggest that IC/BPS with Hunner lesion and IC/BPS without Hunner lesion have different characteristics, and intravesical DMSO treatment with strong anti-inflammatory effects may play a greater role in Hunner lesion type IC/BPS.

2.2 Hyaluronic acid

Hyaluronic acid (HA) is a component of the glycosaminoglycan (GAG) layer of the bladder and is used to repair the GAG layer. A previous study synthesis in an inflammatory model of IC/BPS indicated that the mechanism of action involves modulation of urothelial permeability and stimulation of GAG [10]. HA is used at a concentration of 0.8% for intravesical instillation treatment for IC/BPS. In a previous study in which intravesical HA was administered for 4 weeks with monthly instillation for 6 months in patients with refractory IC/BPS, the response rate at 12 weeks was 71% and was maintained well until 20 weeks. In a study comparing HA and heparin intravesical instillation after hydrodistension, the therapeutic effect of severe IC/BPS patients was maintained longer in patients who received HA instillation than those who received heparin.

2.3 Chondroitin sulfate

Chondroitin sulfate (CS) is a glycoprotein and a component of the GAG layer of bladder mucosa. Commercially available CS products include iAluRil (Juno, AK), Uracyst (Galen, UK), and Uropol (Galen). Nickel et al. [11] performed a multicenter, randomized, double-blind study in which 20 ml of 2% CS or an inactive control solution were injected weekly for 8 weeks for female patients with IC/BPS. The proportion of patients with moderate or marked improvement at 11 weeks was 38.0% in the CS group and 31.3% in the control group; CS treatment in IC/BPS patients showed minor improvements in IC/BPS-related symptom and pain. In another recent report, intravesical CS was found to be superior to intravesical HA in terms of frequency, nocturia and ICPI in patients with BPS/IC during the 6 months of follow-up [12]. In refractory IC/BPS patients, the combination of 1.6% HA and 2.0% CS maintained improvement in symptoms for up to 3 years, indicating that the combination treatment might be more effective than the monotherapy [13].

3. Transurethral surgical ablation

3.1 Symptom control

If a Hunner lesion is confirmed by cystoscopy, transurethral surgical treatment should be performed. In 1971, Kerr et al. [14] first performed transurethral resection on a female patient with Hunner lesion who reported symptom relief for 1 year. In 2000, Peeker et al. [15] reported that 40% of patients who underwent transurethral resection of Hunner lesion had symptomatic improvement; the remission rate was 34.5%, and patients remained in remission for 3 years after resection. In addition, Lee et al. [16] reported that combined hydrodistension and transurethral resection treatment increased bladder capacity and reduced the frequency of micturition and pain. Although the transurethral ablation methods, such as fulguration, coagulation, or resection of Hunner lesion, differ according to various studies, the pain visual analogue scale (VAS) significantly improved after transurethral ablation.

We performed a prospective, observational study of 72 patients with IC/BPS with Hunner lesion who underwent transurethral ablation and followed patients for 3 years [17]. At one month after surgery, the mean number of frequency and mean number of urgency episodes decreased sharply to 5.5 times and 9.4 times, respectively. Over the 12-month follow-up period, the number of frequency, urgency and VAS pain score increased compared with immediately after primary ablation treatment; however, these indices were all significantly better, even after 12 months.

3.2 Characteristics of recurrence

As the extent of Hunner lesion increases, the patient's pain and urinary symptoms tend to become more severe. The ICSI and ICPI and the maximum bladder capacity are significantly associated with the extent of Hunner lesion [18]. Nevertheless, it seems unlikely that patients with multiple Hunner lesion or a wider extent of Hunner lesion are more likely to show recurrence. Akiyama et al. [18] performed hydrodistension with fulguration for Hunner lesion and evaluated the outcome according to the extent of Hunner lesion; the authors found that the extent of Hunner lesion did not predict the need for repeat hydrodistension/fulguration. In our previous study, we were also unable to identify predictive factors related to recurrence. Lower maximal cystometric capacity [odds ratio (OR) 1.01, 95% CI 1.001–1.013; P = 0.017] was the only predictive factor related to early recurrence within 12 months, but sex, presence of previous hydrodistension, and number of Hunner lesions did not affect early recurrence [17]. Han et al. [19] also examined the recurrence pattern and predictors of Hunner lesion; the number of Hunner lesions had no effect on recurrence and only the Pelvic Pain and Urgency/Frequency Patient Symptom Scale (PUF) bother score (OR 1.142, 95% CI 1.016–1.284, P = 0.026) was a predictor related to recurrence of Hunner lesion. A PUF bother score greater than or equal to 7.5 was identified as the predictive cut-off value for recurrence, with a ROC area of 0.690 (sensitivity: 67.9%, specificity: 62.5%). In summary, the predictors of Hunner lesion recurrence have not yet been clearly identified; recurrence or progression does not appear to be faster in patients with multiple Hunner lesions and severe symptoms at the time of initial diagnosis.

One study evaluated the recurrence patterns of Hunner lesion after transurethral ablation and showed that 21.8% of Hunner lesions recurred in the previous ablation site, 18.8% recurred in a de novo site, and 59.4% recurred in both previous and de novo sites [19]. We analyzed the recurrence pattern through prospectively collected data of IC/BPS patients with Hunner lesion who underwent transurethral ablation (data not yet published). In our cases, Hunner lesion recurred in 120 of 210 patients with a median follow-up of 32 months. Among patients with a first recurrence, the proportion of patients with recurrence at the previous ablation site was 50.8% (n = 61), while 6.7% (n = 8) had recurrence of a new lesion, and 42.5% (n = 51) had recurrence at both previous and new sites. Overall, 90% of patients had recurrence around the previous ablation site, and less than 7% showed recurrence at a new site. Endoscopic treatment for Hunner lesion shows good efficacy in alleviating symptoms for a specific period of time after the procedure, but ultimately does not prevent Hunner lesion recurrence. This is considered a natural course of IC/BPS with

Hunner lesion disease with the characteristics of pancystitis. To prevent recurrence, the role of postoperative medication or intravesical treatment should be investigated. A recent pilot study reported that hydrodistension with fulguration of Hunner lesion plus maintenance DMSO therapy prolonged the recurrence-free time in patients with IC/BPS with Hunner lesion [20].

3.3 Does repeat treatment reduce recurrence?

One question regarding the recurrence of Hunner lesions is whether endoscopic treatment helps to suppress recurrence. However, current research indicates this may not be the case. In a 30-month prospective study of IC/BPS with Hunner lesion treatment naïve patients, the median recurrence-free time after the first endoscopic ablation of Hunner lesion was 12.0 ± 1.6 months (95% CI; 8.9–15.1). After the second endoscopic ablation, the median recurrence-free time was 18.0 ± 5.1 months (95% CI; 8.0–28.0), which was slightly increased, but the difference was not statistically significant ($p = 0.15$) [17]. Nevertheless, if Hunner lesion recurs, repeat ablation should be performed. Repeated endoscopic ablation does not lower the recurrence rate, but it is the only way to significantly reduce pain and improve quality of life in a less invasive manner.

3.4 Which endoscopic treatment, transurethral resection or coagulation, can further reduce recurrence?

Prominent ulcerations are observed in the histology of Hunner lesion, which may be covered by fibrin mixed with inflammatory cells, in particular neutrophils. The lesions are often wedge-shaped and involve the superficial part of the lamina propria, often extending into the muscularis mucosae. Thus, deep biopsies including bladder muscle are required, since the disease process involves superficial as well as deeper layers of the bladder wall [4]. Many symptoms and findings in IC/BPS with Hunner lesion may be ascribed to the release of mast cell–derived factors. Mast cells are often observed near nerves, and functional evidence suggests innervation of these cells. As a hypothesis that has been accepted so far, transurethral ablation might be the removal of intramural nerve endings engaged in the inflammatory process [21–23].

Whether transurethral resection of Hunner lesion is capable of disease control compared with coagulation/fulguration and prevents recurrence of Hunner lesion is an important question. A randomized controlled study was conducted to compare the therapeutic effect between transurethral resection and coagulation of Hunner lesion in 126 patients with IC/BPS [24]. The primary endpoint was the difference in recurrence-free time between the two surgical methods, and the secondary outcomes were voiding symptoms, pain level, and risk factors for recurrence. The median duration of follow-up was 11.0 months. There were no differences in the recurrence-free time between the treatment groups: 12.2 months (95% confidence interval [CI], 11.1–17.6) for the transurethral resection group and 11.5 months (95% CI, 9.03–16.1; $p = 0.735$) for the transurethral coagulation group. In addition, after both procedures, the mean daytime frequency, nocturia, urgency episodes, ICSI, ICPI, PUF symptom scale, and VAS for pain all improved significantly compared with baseline; however, there were no differences between the groups over 12 months. The type of surgery, age, number of Hunner lesions, and maximal cystomteric capacity were not associated with the risk of recurrence. In safety analysis, in cases treated with transurethral resection, the incidence of bladder injury was 7.9%, which was slightly higher than that among patients treated with coagulation, which was 3.4%. Our findings did not suggest that one procedure was superior to the other with regard to delaying recurrence. The choice of treatment did not affect the recurrence rate and produced comparable results, which may be because the ultimate peripheral denervation acted as the same thermal effect in both treatments.

3.5 Is it helpful to perform concurrent hydrodistension before transurethral ablation?

Some studies have suggested that concurrent hydrodistension with transurethral ablation may be helpful for symptom improvement [16, 18, 25]. However, the simultaneous performance of hydrodistension causes difficulties in complete removal of the Hunner lesion. Hydrodistension obscures the boundaries of the Hunner lesion, which are clearly identified through cystoscopy, and bleeding related to hydrodistension interferes with the field of surgical view. We believe that good efficacy can be maintained only with transurethral resection or coagulation of Hunner lesion without hydrodistension.

3.6 Technique of transurethral coagulation and resection of Hunner lesion

To coagulate or resect the Hunner lesion, the most important first step is to demarcate the lesion with the cautery before full bladder distension. Complete coagulation of the inside Hunner lesion of the boundary should then be performed. If starting from the inside of the lesion and working outward, reactive erythema spreads outward and obscures the original boundary of the lesion. In the case of transurethral resection, it is effective to use a bipolar loop. During the resection, resection should be performed as deeply as possible to the muscle layer using a cutting current. However, bladder damage can easily occur because the bladder wall of Hunner lesion is thin and friable. To prevent bladder injury, the quantity of irrigation fluid should be kept constant through suction attached to the outer sheath. Using this approach, the risk of bladder damage can be reduced by preventing the overdistension of bladder. Nevertheless, when it is difficult to complete resect the Hunner lesion or when the surgeon does not have extensive experience for transurethral resection, transurethral coagulation alone may be enough to control Hunner lesions.

4. Reconstructive surgery

Partial or complete cystectomy, augmentation cystoplasty, and urinary diversion are options indicated by the AUA and East Asian guidelines when all other therapies have failed [1, 7]. Rossberger et al. [26] found that reconstructive surgery resulted in the resolution of symptoms in 94% of patients with refractory IC/BPS with Hunner lesion. Patients with IC/BPS with Hunner lesion had a significantly smaller bladder capacity and benefited from reconstructive surgery compared with patients without Hunner lesion. We retrospectively analyzed 40 patients who underwent augmentation ileocystoplasty with supratrigonal cystectomy in patients with refractory IC/BPS with Hunner lesion [27]. After augmentation with supratrigonal cystectomy, significantly decreased pain and frequency and significantly increased bladder capacity were observed. Treatment failure was defined as the persistence of symptoms after surgery or a less than 30% reduction in ICSI from baseline, which accounted for 20% (8/40) of patients. Two of the patients had recurrent Hunner lesion around the bladder neck and additional endoscopic ablation was performed, while the remaining patients maintained oral medication [27].

There may be concerns about major complications after reconstructive surgery; however, most complications were minor and managed conservatively. Although six patients had vesicoureteral reflux after surgery, there was no deterioration of the upper urinary tract, so no additional treatment was required. Five patients received intermittent catheterization because they were unable to void after surgery, but the discomfort of catheterization was not considered a significant problem due to improvement in pain [27].

5. Conclusion

Although there is no definite treatment for IC/BPS, endoscopic treatment can be considered for Hunner lesion type IC/BPS. To confirm the presence of Hunner lesion, cystoscopy should be performed in patients with suspected IC/BPS. When performing cystoscopy, the bladder should not be inflated too much to prevent false-positive findings or bleeding due to mucosal fissure and to accurately diagnose Hunner lesion. Various intravesical therapies, including HA, CS, and DMSO, have been used for IC/BPS and are more effective in terms of anti-inflammatory effects and GAG layer replenishment in patients with Hunner lesion than patients without Hunner lesion. Overall, endoscopic ablation for Hunner lesion is an effective and minimally invasive treatment for patients with Hunner lesion type IC/BPS; this treatment strategy significantly reduces pain and improves voiding symptoms. Mucosal cracks that occur during hydrodistension are not real Hunner lesion, and we do not recommend performing hydrodistension first during endoscopic ablation. Repeated ablation does not suppress recurrence but does not reduce the therapeutic efficacy. There are various methods for endoscopic ablation; the main methods are coagulation or resection of Hunner lesion, and both are good treatment modalities to relieve the symptoms of Hunner lesion IC/BPS and improve quality of life. IC/BPS with Hunner lesion is a progressive disease, and it is necessary to establish a treatment protocol such as adjuvant intravesical treatment to reduce the risk of recurrence after transurethral ablation.

Author details

Kwang Jin Ko[1] and Kyu-Sung Lee[1,2]*

1 Department of Urology, Samsung Medical Center, Sungkyunkwan University School of Medicine, Seoul, Republic of Korea

2 Research Institute for Future Medicine Samsung Medical Center, Seoul, Korea

*Address all correspondence to: ksleedr@skku.edu

References

[1] Homma Y, Akiyama Y, Tomoe H, et al. Clinical guidelines for interstitial cystitis/bladder pain syndrome. Int J Urol 2020;27:578-89.

[2] Whitmore KE, Fall M, Sengiku A, Tomoe H, Logadottir Y, Kim YH. Hunner lesion versus non-Hunner lesion interstitial cystitis/bladder pain syndrome. Int J Urol 2019;26 Suppl 1:26-34.

[3] Maeda D, Akiyama Y, Morikawa T, et al. Hunner-Type (Classic) Interstitial Cystitis: A Distinct Inflammatory Disorder Characterized by Pancystitis, with Frequent Expansion of Clonal B-Cells and Epithelial Denudation. PLoS One 2015;10:e0143316.

[4] Fall M, Nordling J, Cervigni M, et al. Hunner lesion disease differs in diagnosis, treatment and outcome from bladder pain syndrome: an ESSIC working group report. Scand J Urol 2020;54:91-8.

[5] Lai HH, Pickersgill NA, Vetter JM. Hunner Lesion Phenotype in Interstitial Cystitis/Bladder Pain Syndrome: A Systematic Review and Meta-Analysis. J Urol 2020;204:518-23.

[6] Rawls WF, Cox L, Rovner ES. Dimethyl sulfoxide (DMSO) as intravesical therapy for interstitial cystitis/bladder pain syndrome: A review. Neurourol Urodyn 2017;36: 1677-84.

[7] Hanno PM, Erickson D, Moldwin R, Faraday MM. Diagnosis and treatment of interstitial cystitis/bladder pain syndrome: AUA guideline amendment. J Urol 2015;193:1545-53.

[8] Perez-Marrero R, Emerson LE, Feltis JT. A controlled study of dimethyl sulfoxide in interstitial cystitis. J Urol 1988;140:36-9.

[9] Yoshimura N, Homma Y, Tomoe H, et al. Efficacy and safety of intravesical instillation of KRP-116D (50% dimethyl sulfoxide solution) for interstitial cystitis/bladder pain syndrome in Japanese patients: A multicenter, randomized, double-blind, placebo-controlled, clinical study. Int J Urol 2021;28:545-53.

[10] Rooney P, Srivastava A, Watson L, Quinlan LR, Pandit A. Hyaluronic acid decreases IL-6 and IL-8 secretion and permeability in an inflammatory model of interstitial cystitis. Acta Biomater 2015;19:66-75.

[11] Nickel JC, Hanno P, Kumar K, Thomas H. Second multicenter, randomized, double-blind, parallel-group evaluation of effectiveness and safety of intravesical sodium chondroitin sulfate compared with inactive vehicle control in subjects with interstitial cystitis/bladder pain syndrome. Urology 2012;79:1220-4.

[12] Gülpınar Ö, Esen B, Kayış A, Gökçe M, Süer E. Clinical comparison of intravesical hyaluronic acid and chondroitin sulfate therapies in the treatment of bladder pain syndrome/ interstitial cystitis. Neurourol Urodyn 2018;37:257-62.

[13] Cervigni M, Natale F, Nasta L, Mako A. Intravesical hyaluronic acid and chondroitin sulphate for bladder pain syndrome/interstitial cystitis: long-term treatment results. Int Urogynecol J 2012;23:1187-92.

[14] Kerr WS, Jr. Interstitial cystitis: treatment by transurethral resection. J Urol 1971;105:664-6.

[15] Peeker R, Aldenborg F, Fall M. Complete transurethral resection of ulcers in classic interstitial cystitis. Int Urogynecol J Pelvic Floor Dysfunct 2000;11:290-5.

[16] Lee ES, Lee SW, Lee KW, Kim JM, Kim YH, Kim ME. Effect of

transurethral resection with hydrodistention for the treatment of ulcerative interstitial cystitis. Korean J Urol 2013;54:682-8.

[17] Ko KJ, Chung H, Suh YS, Lee SW, Kim TH, Lee KS. Therapeutic effects of endoscopic ablation in patients with Hunner type interstitial cystitis. BJU Int 2018;121:659-66.

[18] Akiyama Y, Niimi A, Nomiya A, et al. Extent of Hunner lesions: The relationships with symptom severity and clinical parameters in Hunner type interstitial cystitis patients. Neurourol Urodyn 2018;37:1441-7.

[19] Han JY, Shin JH, Choo MS. Patterns and predictors of Hunner lesion recurrence in patients with interstitial cystitis. Neurourol Urodyn 2019;38:1392-8.

[20] Otsuka A, Suzuki T, Matsushita Y, et al. Therapeutic Endoscopic Treatment Plus Maintenance Dimethyl Sulfoxide Therapy Prolongs Recurrence-Free Time in Patients With Hunner Type Interstitial Cystitis: A Pilot Study. Int Neurourol J 2019;23:327-33.

[21] Kim HJ. Update on the Pathology and Diagnosis of Interstitial Cystitis/ Bladder Pain Syndrome: A Review. Int Neurourol J 2016;20:13-7.

[22] Fall M. Conservative management of chronic interstitial cystitis: transcutaneous electrical nerve stimulation and transurethral resection. J Urol 1985;133:774-8.

[23] Newson B, Dahlström A, Enerbäck L, Ahlman H. Suggestive evidence for a direct innervation of mucosal mast cells. Neuroscience 1983;10:565-70.

[24] Ko KJ, Cho WJ, Lee YS, Choi J, Byun HJ, Lee KS. Comparison of the Efficacy Between Transurethral Coagulation and Transurethral Resection of Hunner Lesion in Interstitial Cystitis/Bladder Pain Syndrome Patients: A Prospective Randomized Controlled Trial. Eur Urol 2020;77:644-51.

[25] Chennamsetty A, Khourdaji I, Goike J, Killinger KA, Girdler B, Peters KM. Electrosurgical management of Hunner ulcers in a referral center's interstitial cystitis population. Urology 2015;85:74-8.

[26] Rössberger J, Fall M, Jonsson O, Peeker R. Long-term results of reconstructive surgery in patients with bladder pain syndrome/interstitial cystitis: subtyping is imperative. Urology 2007;70:638-42.

[27] Kim HJ, Lee JS, Cho WJ, et al. Efficacy and safety of augmentation ileocystoplasty combined with supratrigonal cystectomy for the treatment of refractory bladder pain syndrome/interstitial cystitis with Hunner's lesion. Int J Urol 2014;21 Suppl 1:69-73.

Chapter 6

Development of Management Model Post-Stroke Urinary Incontinence

Heltty Heltty, Ratna Sitorus, Nury Nusdwinuringtyas and Evi Martha

Abstract

Post-stroke urinary incontinence (UI) is one of the sequelae of stroke. This situation affects all aspects of the patient's life both physically, psychologically, socially, and spiritually. Post-stroke UI as a chronic disease requires holistic treatment. Many chronic health problems will respond well when handled from a holistic perspective. The holistic health view focuses on the patient's health care needs, not only needs related to the patient's physical condition of health, but also subjective aspects related to social representation of his/her health conditions. Developing a holistic post-stroke UI management model and continuous care at the patient's home needs to be done. This chapter includes model components which are also interventions that can be done to overcome post-stroke UI. These interventions include information and understanding of post-stroke UI; ways to overcome post-stroke UI; conduct self-control and stay motivated; perform daily activities independently according to ability; and get family support and peer attention. This model was developed based on previous qualitative studies and literature studies related to post-stroke urinary incontinence. Intervention in this model is aimed at patients who have passed the acute phase of stroke, when they will be discharge from the hospital and continued at the patient's home.

Keywords: Post-stroke urinary incontinence, holistic care, continuous care, hospitalized, patient's home, intervention model

1. Introduction

Urinary Incontinence (UI) is characterized by involuntary leakage of urine, which can occur immediately after a stroke or later [1]. The prevalence of post-stroke UI ranges from 32% - 79%, of which approximately 25% - 28% of patients experienced UI after discharged from the hospital and about 15% experienced UI one year after discharged from hospital [2]. The incidence of post-stroke UI in patients older than 75 years old was higher than in patients aged less than 75 years [3]. International studies showed the average prevalence of UI was 8.2% to 26.8% in 2016, of which 13% - 38.7% occurred in women and 2.9% - 9.9% in men. When compared with the elderly population, the prevalence of UI in the elderly reached an average of 29.4% where 26.7% - 36.3% of this number occurred in women and 6.4% - 17% in men [4].

Post-stroke UI affects all aspect of a person's life (physically, psychologically, socially, and spiritually), so that it situation affects the patient's quality of life [5–8]. Research has found that 66% of UI on women report that their quality of life was affected by their UI [8]. Post-stroke UI is also associated with limb weakness that prevents patients from urinating in the toilet. Post-stroke UI patients need a management post-stroke urinary incontinence in a holistic and continuous care manner up to the patient's home so as to increase the patient's independence. Therefore, the basic theories used in developing this model are the Human becoming theory, the Self-care deficit theory of nursing, and several theories related to post-stroke UI.

The critical point in this model is the development of management model post-stroke urinary incontinence in a holistic and continuous care manner up to the patient's home which is developed through up-to-date justification to describe what things are need to do in this model as an effort to improve patient independence.

2. Model description

This post-stroke UI management model is a model of post-stroke UI management in nursing that is carried out holistically and given by nurses to stroke patients who have UI and have passed the acute period of stroke. It begins when the patient will go out from hospital and continuing at the patient's home. Implementation of the model begins with the nurse identifying the patient's health condition, including identifying the patient's performance status using the Karnofsky scale, and monitoring the patient's incontinence status using the Bladder diary format for three days (72 hours). After that, the nurse and the patient together determine the goals to be achieved using the SMART method (specific, measurable, achievable, realistic, and there is a time limit).

The implementation of the post-stroke UI management model includes providing information and understanding about post-stroke UI, ways to deal with post-stroke UI, self-control and staying motivated, performing daily activities independently according to patient's ability, and increasing family support and peer attention.

Providing information and understanding about post-stroke UI through health education about post-stroke UI which includes definition, etiology, pathophysiology, types of post-stroke UI, assessment of post-stroke UI, and treatment of post-stroke UI. Increasing the patient's ability to perform ways to deal with post-stroke UI is also through health education and skills training such as bladder retraining, pelvic floor muscle exercise, deep breathing relaxation exercise, and range of motion (ROM) exercise. Self-control and staying motivated also through health education about positive thinking and controlling emotions. Carrying out daily activities independently according to ability is carried out gradually involving patients in daily activities at home such as activities related to personal hygiene and household chores. Family support in every action taken by the patient and the involvement of peers who have successfully overcome post-stroke UI in sharing experiences about things that have been done while experiencing post-stroke UI. In the final stage of model, the nurse evaluates and conveys the results of the evaluation of the achievement of goals to the patient.

3. Model development process

This post-stroke UI management model was developed based on literature studies, result of previous qualitative research, and expert consultation. The integration of theories used to develop this model is described in detail as follows:

3.1 Post-stroke urinary incontinence

3.1.1 Definition of post-stroke urinary incontinence

Post-stroke Urinary Incontinence (UI) is an involuntary (unconscious) leakage of urine, which can occur immediately after a stroke or later [1]. UI is a condition that affects the physical and psychological aspects of life with consequences that affect the quality of life [9]. UI has been shown to disrupt patients and negatively affect many aspects of life, including sleep quality, emotional well-being and depression, social relationships, work productivity, and overall health-related quality of life. The symptoms of urinary disorders can affect daily routines, causing limitations in physical, social, occupational, domestic, and sexual activities. Post-stroke UI interferes with the patient's activities of daily living and social activities so that it can lead to a reduced desire to participate in the treatment program [10]. Social and hygienic discomfort caused by the fear of passing urine and the smell of urine, can affect the quality of life. UI patients were burdened with anxiety, feelings of shame, and they live in fear that others will discover their condition. Major depression has been shown to add to a cycle of low self-esteem, increased social withdrawal, and ultimately decreased quality of life [11].

3.1.2 Types of post-stroke urinary incontinence and their causes

The types of post-stroke UI and their causes can be seen in **Table 1**:

3.1.3 Pathophysiology of post-stroke urinary incontinence

Damage to the midbrain that responsible for micturition can result in an inability to coordinate bladder contractions with urethral sphincter relaxation. After a stroke, the brain may enter a transient phase of acute brain shock. During this time, the bladder will be in retention – detrusor areflexia. After the brain shock phase subsides, the bladder exhibits detrusor hyperreflexia (overactivity of the bladder detrusor) with coordinated urethral sphincter activity. This occurs because the pontine micturition center (PMC) is responsible for suppressing the periaqueductal

Types of post-stroke urinary incontinence	Causes of post-stroke urinary incontinence
Detrusor hyperreflexia and urge incontinence	Direct damage to the neuromicturation pathway; Accidental leakage of urine accompanied or preceded by urgency
Detrusor hyporeflexia and overflow incontinence	Loss of bladder tone and non-stroke factors; Continuous dribbling and/or leakage of urine with incomplete bladder emptying and urinary retention
Awareness of urinary incontinence is impaired	Reduced ability to be aware of bladder signals before a leak, to notice a possible leak, or both
Functional incontinence	Communicative, cognitive, and mobility impairments causing UI despite normal bladder function.
Stress incontinence	Not directly due to a stroke but pre-existing problems can make things worse. Stress incontinence occurs when the urethral sphincter, pelvic floor muscles, or both of these structures have weakened or been damaged so that they cannot hold urine continuously.

Table 1.
Types of post-stroke urinary incontinence and their causes.

gray (PAG) which is located in the midbrain and directs the urethral sphincter and bladder wall muscle activity to maintain bladder control, cause the weakening of these processes [12]. When the pontine is damaged by a stroke, hyperreflexia of the detrusor muscle can occur, causing symptoms of "frequency" and "urge" to urinate [13]. Sensation of urinary urgency is characterized by more frequent micturition throughout the day and night [14].

3.1.4 Characteristics of post-stroke urinary incontinence

Cerebellar stroke patients' urodynamically more frequently reported signs of detrusor overactivity (53–77%), external detrusor sphincter dyssinergy (40%), and inability to relax the urinary sphincter (47%) [1]. Urge incontinence is characterized by a person who has a strong urge to urinate suddenly followed by involuntary urination (wetting the bed), the frequency of urinating more than 8 times a day, including at night. Stress incontinence is characterized by urine leaking out when there is pressure on the bladder, for example when coughing, sneezing, or laughing. Stress incontinence often precedes stroke symptoms but is usually exacerbated after stroke with recurrent coughing associated with dysphagia and aspiration [15]. Functional incontinence usually occurs in patients who are aware of the need to urinate but have functional limitations to reach the toilet [1].

3.1.5 Assessment of post-stroke urinary incontinence

The assessment can be started with identifying the patient's health condition, including identifying the patient's performance status using the Karnofsky scale, and monitoring the patient's incontinence status using the Bladder diary format for three days (72 hours). Physical assessment and history-taking, including identification of urological problems before the stroke occurred such as bladder outlet obstruction or stress incontinence [16]. Physical assessment also including pain, haematuria, history of recurrent urinary tract infection (UTI), pelvic surgery, and UI associated with known abnormality of the urinary tract [17]. Careful abdominal examination should be performed, an abdominal mass can contribute to stress incontinence and occasionally can cause urinary obstruction with resultant overflow incontinence. The cough test should be performed with the full bladder comfortably in a standing position and it may reveal SUI. In neurologic patients, evaluation of lower extremity strength, reflexes and perineal sensation is necessary. Unilateral weakness or hyperreflexia of the lower extremities may identify an upper motor lesion [17].

In addition, it is also necessary to assessment onset and duration of symptoms, urgency, dribbling, symptoms related to a specific activity such as coughing, sneezing. Assessment of pre-existing incontinence, associated bowel symptoms, medication such as diuretic, anticholinergic, oestrogens, sedatives, and antidepressants. Assessment about fluid intake; medical history related to diabetes, recurrent urinary tract infections and dementia; cognitive ability; and functional capacity: dexterity, mobility, and aids [10].

3.1.6 Management of post-stroke urinary incontinence

There are several successful options for controlling UI, including: nursing interventions in the form of behavioral therapy, pharmacological agents, and surgical treatments [18]. Behavioral treatments are recommended as the first therapy for UI management [1, 19]. It is also recommended by the Intercollegiate Stroke Working Party (2012) and the National Institute for Health and Care Excellence

(2012). Based on the recommendations of the Agency for Health Policy and Research Guidelines (APCHR) and the International Consultation on Incontinence that UI intervention is at least invasive, behavioral management should be initiated early [15].

Behavioral treatment (include bladder retraining and pelvic floor muscle training) can improve bladder control by changing urinary habits experienced by UI patients and teach skills to prevent urine leakage [20]. Several studies mention that the effectiveness of bladder retraining and pelvic floor muscle training in treating UI. There are several advantages of behavioral intervention, including the absence of side effects, comfort, and patient satisfaction [20].

These behavioral interventions need to be taught by nurses to post-stroke UI patients. Families as caregivers also need to be involved in the care of post-stroke UI patients. Management of post-stroke UI needs support family and friends [21]. Families can provide support in the form of emotional and instrumental support by motivating and facilitating patients in providing the necessary equipment such as walking aids and supporting patient healing, including physical support in the form of providing time to assist patients in the management of post-stroke UI. Support from friends can help reduce feeling of isolation and fear, where support from friends who have also experienced in the same diseases can be done by sharing experiences and providing information about necessary health services [22]. Patients are also involved in daily activities so that they can improve the patient's ability and reduce anxiety, where anxiety can also affect UI. Anxiety can directly affect bladder function, this leads to changes in bladder pressure [23]. Changes in bladder pressure can be characterized by abnormal function and condition of the lower urinary tract due to over activity of the bladder wall muscles that cause a sudden urge to urinate [24].

Previous research has shown that supportive care in cancer patients can improve their mood, reduce anxiety, and reduce depression in patients [25]. Supportive interventions also provide ongoing benefits in reducing depressive symptoms in dementia patients [26]. Supportive interventions increase patient satisfaction, significantly reduce depressive symptoms, and improve quality of life [27]. Peer support can help reduce feeling of isolation and fear, where peer support can be done by sharing experiences and providing information about necessary health services [22].

3.2 Relationship between human becoming theory and post-stroke UI

The theory of human becoming was developed by Rosemarie Parse. Parse views human, the universe, and health as inseparable, irreducible, and ever-changing [28]. Humans are an integral part of the environment, which is constantly changing and evolving with the environment. This provides a perspective that although healing is subjective, environmental factors are essentially a part of, can influence, and may facilitate the healing process. Nurses can help to create a healing environment for patients and families, by being with them and having the intention to be partners in patient care, respecting, and exploring subjective elements that can facilitate mind, body, and spirit healing [29].

Post-stroke UI patients require holistic and sustainable care in manner up to the patient's home. The holistic care model provides support to humans and focuses not only on completing the task of caring for physical aspects of the patient's chronic illness but also the human soul [30]. A holistic approach to nursing as a process strengthens every system of the human mind–body and allows natural healing potentials to develop. Many chronic health problems will respond well if handled from a holistic perspective [31].

Humans as bio-psycho-social-spiritual beings form meaning from previous experiences. The meaning associated with this experience reflects their personal values which are grown through powering and shows the individual's uniqueness in improving the quality of his/her life that needs to be maintained and improved. All aspects of human health, including quality of life, are determined by physical, chemical, biological, social, and psychological factors in the environment. Healing involves being open to one's presence as well as the environment. Emotional, physical, and spiritual closeness is needed in providing care to post-stroke UI patients.

3.3 Relationship between self-care deficit theory of nursing and post-stroke UI

Self-care deficit theory of nursing was developed by Dorothea Elizabeth Orem. In Orem's theory, humans are viewed as agents with the potential for power to satisfy their own needs for self-care. Self-care is not limited to people providing care for them, but also includes care offered by others such as nurses, and/or family members. In Orem's theory, it is explained that humans have the ability to care for themselves and if this ability is distorted by a person, then nurses help individuals to regain their self-care abilities by providing direct care and support through health education. One of the main elements of self-care is health education to patients. Health education helps patients to do self-care because self-care requires the ability to treat them. The need for care exists when the demand for self-care exceeds the capabilities of the self-care agent. Nurses act as facilitators and change agents who can teach how to solve problems and make decisions regarding self-care.

Self-care must be learned and must be done deliberately. Self-care behavior is influenced by the total skills and knowledge that a person has and uses for his/her practical efforts. Self-care is considered an important and valuable principle because it emphasizes an active role in their own health care, not a passive one [32]. Post-stroke UI patients need skills training to overcome their UI. These exercise include bladder retraining, pelvic floor muscle exercise, and ROM. Individual/patients who do pelvic floor exercise must have confidence and be motivated to do exercises regularly despite obstacles or difficulties in daily life [33]. Bladder retraining requires patients to be independent and motivated to participate actively in treatment [34].

The results of observations during previous research, respondent who actively did ROM showed their involvement in caring out daily activities such as helping with housework, fulfilling their needs related to personal hygiene such as bathing, dressing, and starting to be able to walk to urinate in the toilet so that the quality of life respondents the intervention group related to UI slowly showed improvement. These observations were in line with other studies that daily activity training could improve quality of life [35].

3.4 Overview of the results of a qualitative study of patients' experience success in dealing with post-stroke UI

The results of our qualitative study on the patient's experience of successfully dealing with post-stroke UI were also used as a basis for developing a management model post-stroke urinary incontinence in a holistic and continuous care manner up to the patient's home The resulting themes are: (1) Information and understanding about post-stroke UI, (2) Performing ways to deal with post-stroke UI, (3) Self-control and staying motivated, (4) Performing daily activities independently according to patients' ability, and (5) Family support and peer's attention. The results of this thematic analysis are integrated with the human becoming theory, self-care deficit theory of nursing, and other theories related to post-stroke UI. This qualitative study uses an applied qualitative research design with the type of research Rapid Assessment Procedure (RAP). RAP is used as a method to interact directly to discuss or listen to what experiences the patient has had during post-stroke UI. In-depth interviews were used by researchers to obtain daily experiences of patients during post-stroke UI. The in-depth interview guide was developed based on the human becoming theory and the self-care deficit theory of nursing [36].

4. Model schematic

The patient's independence in dealing with post-stroke UI is at the core of the problem regarding the need to provide information and understanding about post-stroke UI, perform ways to deal with post-stroke UI, perform self-control and staying motivated, perform daily activities independently according to patient's ability, and get family support and peer's attention. The schema of the post-stroke UI management model that we developed which is shown in **Figure 1**.

5. Model component

This model includes five components in managing post-stroke UI, namely 1) Improving the provision of information and understanding about post-stroke UI, 2) Improving the ability to do ways to deal with post-stroke UI, 3) Improving self-control and staying motivated, 4) Improving ability carry out activities independently according to patient's ability, and 5) Improving family support and peer's attention in managing post-stroke UI. The following described the components of this model in more detail:

5.1 Improving the provision of information and understanding of post-stroke UI

The basis for implementing this theme is the finding of our previous qualitative study which showed that informants (patients) need information to increase their knowledge in recognizing and understanding various physical and psychosocial conditions that occur to them. This information can make it easier for patients to overcome problems related to post-stroke UI that they were experiencing.

Information is provided through health education about post-stroke UI which includes an explanation of the basic concepts of post-stroke UI such as definition, causes, the process of occurrence, signs and symptoms that appear, types of post-stroke UI, and how to deal with post-stroke UI. Nurses need to build a trusting relationship and conduct an initial assessment of the patient's knowledge regarding the patient's perceived physical and psychosocial conditions.

Providing education about post-stroke UI is given to patients and their families as caregivers. Before educating patient and caregivers, nurses seek information from patients related to what patients have known about post-stroke UI. This makes it easier for nurses to provide further information. Information from patients is a central aspect of patient-centered care [37]. The information conveyed by the patient reflects the patient's knowledge about their condition [38]. Nurses have the potential to identify people with incontinence, establish appropriate interventions, and provide valuable health education to empower patients [39]. Providing information related to a through assessment in describing the type and severity of incontinence is needed to provide treatment/nursing care according to individual needs [10].

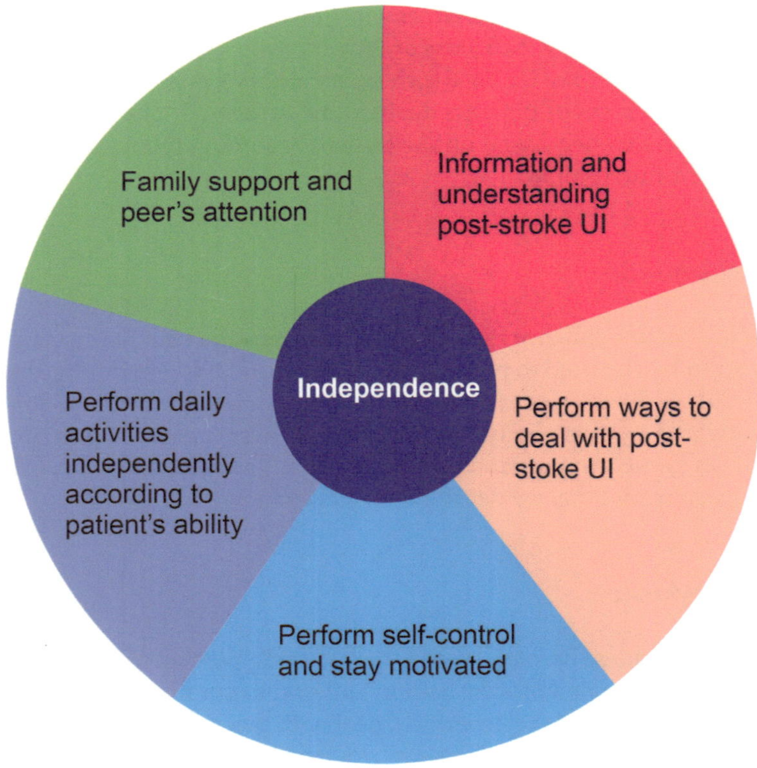

Figure 1.
Model schema of post-stroke urinary incontinence management.

Post-stroke UI is a taboo subject in society; patient openness in providing information to nurses is very much needed. In an effort to increase patient openness, there needs to be a trusting relationship between patients and nurses. In-depth interviews that researchers conducted in digging up information related to post-stroke UI were not easy to do. Some informants did not immediately open up if they had experienced UI but by starting questions to explore information related to daily activities, the obstacles found by the patient in carrying out daily activities so that the patient was open to provide information about his current condition.

5.2 Improving the ability to do ways to deal with post-stroke UI

This action needs to be done in management of post-stroke UI. The results of our qualitative study showed that the informants/patients did several ways to overcome their post-stroke UI such as bladder retraining, pelvic floor muscle exercises, distraction technique, and ROM exercises. These ways describe the knowledge, skills, and ability to decide what the patient should do in dealing with his illness. Based on these findings, it appears that the patient is not only focused on improving the functional ability to urinate but also improving the functional ability to walk. In dealing with post-stroke UI, patients need to be trained to improve the functional ability to urinate as well as the functional ability to walk [16].

Such exercises can be provided through health education and demonstrations to patients and caregivers. Skills exercises taught to patients and caregivers include bladder retraining, pelvic floor muscle exercises, and deep breathing relaxation exercises to divert the urge to urinate. In addition, ROM exercises are also done to train the patient's muscle strength so that it can help the patient walk to urinate in the bathroom. Patients and caregivers are given the opportunity to practice and demonstrate the skills that have been taught independently, but are still given continuous supervision to achieve the goals that have been set. This education and skills training can be provided in the hospital after the patient has passed the acute phase of stroke and then continued at the patient's home.

Continental training begins as soon as the patient's condition stabilizes. It is also important to prevent incontinence which may be reversible [1]. Bladder retraining requires that patients be independent and motivated to actively participate in treatment [34]. Bladder retraining trains the patient to empty the bladder at regular intervals. Emptying the bladder at regular time intervals in post-stroke UI patients is a more effective method for treating incontinence [1].

Consider that there is strong evidence that bladder retraining with urge suppression is effective in treating urge incontinence, stress incontinence, and mixed incontinence in adult women. Bladder retraining exercise is also often combined with pelvic floor muscle training (detrusor contraction inhibition) in adults with UI without neurologic disease. This exercise has been shown to be effective in reducing incontinence episodes for three months, compared to bladder retraining with urge suppression alone [34]. Pelvic floor muscle exercises seek to reduce uncontrolled detrusor muscle contractions in patients with better cognitive abilities. Individuals/patients who perform pelvic floor muscle exercises must have confidence and be motivated to perform exercises regularly despite obstacles or difficulties in daily life [33].

Before starting pelvic floor muscle training, it is necessary to ensure that the patient can perform pelvic floor muscle contractions. More than 30% of patients are unable to contract the pelvic floor muscles at the first meeting of educational exercises [40]. So that training and education repeatedly need to be done. Patients and caregivers are also encouraged to always pay attention to environmental conditions, avoid wet floors, pay attention to room lighting during exercise, including eating nutritious foods, and avoiding drinks containing alcohol and caffeine such as tea, coffee, and cola especially before bedtime. Also avoid drinking too little because it can make the urine color dark and can irritate the bladder. Avoid drinking too much and too fast. Advise the patient to drink 500 milliliters at each meal and 200 milliliters between meals, and to drink more fluids in the morning and evening.

The ways that patients do in dealing with post-stroke IU describe the patient's ability and skills to achieve healing. This is based on the knowledge and desire of the patient to recover, so that the patients carry out the process of transferring (transformation) health patterns with the choice to change attitudes in living daily life. In human becoming theory, it is stated that the transformation of health patterns can occur when individuals find insights about themselves that were previously unclear, when they find ways to change towards the hopes and dreams they cherish [28, 41]. The hope for recovery makes the patients always do ways to overcome the post-stroke UI and become the patient's strength when facing the post-stroke UI.

5.3 Improving self-control and stay motivated

Self-control is the inhibiting force that enables the person to adjust decisions and behavior towards long-term targets [42]. Self-control describes how a person chooses and finds ways to deal with the situations they experience. This relates to the values of beliefs held. In Human becoming theory, it is stated that beliefs reflect what is important in a person's life regarding his health, which is the basic for a person to make choices about how to think, act, and feel [43].

Self-control is done by thinking positively and controlling emotions [36]. Positive thinking is done by cultivating positive thoughts, eliminating the burden of thinking about the disease, getting closer to God, and growing belief in healing, including belief related to spirituality in interpreting post-stroke UI [36]. Patients are always reminded of the goals to be achieved and focus on achieving these goals. The success of self-control can be seen in increasing physical activity, improving general health, feeling happy, increasing physical and emotional roles. Positive thinking can be used to improve the quality of live [44]. Other studies have shown that self-control training has a significant effect in improving the quality of life in patients with migraine [42] and improving the quality of life of asthma patients [45].

Positive thinking is the practice or result of a firm mind about what is constructive and about something good, so that it can eliminate negative thoughts and emotions [46]. Positive thinking helps to know and understand self-concept better, and helps to see yourself better. Positive thinking is very important in achieving goals and making a person constructive and creative. Positive thinkers face situations optimistically and if they face stressful situations, then they judge it to be controllable and use coping strategies that are functional, efficient, and problem-focused [47].

Positive thinking is supported by internal cognition, beliefs, and relationships [46]. Beliefs including religious beliefs can help a person cope with a state of uncertainty, including in dealing with stressful life events [48]. Positive thinking is also associated with optimism, perception, and self-esteem [46].

Based on this, the interventions/steps that need to be taken to increase positive thinking include:

- Education to improve patient understanding: explain to patients that inappropriate view or perceptions and attitudes can affect perceptions of urinary incontinence.

- Assist patients in determining treatment goal

- Encourage the patient to pay attention to every thought that is written. Instruct the patient to ask himself whether the thought makes sense?

- Performing distraction techniques includes: using negative thought-stopping techniques (such as focusing on yours surroundings or putting a rubber band on your wrist, scheduling time for rethinking, writing down troublesome thoughts), including diverting attention away from urinating e.g. watching television, reading newspapers, dhikr, reading scriptures, playing games, listening to music, counting backwards, and so on.

- Instruct the patient to meet with other people.

- Patient motivation in achieving their goals, thinking that there are still many other patients who have more severe problems.

- Advise patient to always be optimistic.

- Involve family or loved ones

- Involve local religious leaders to increase patient beliefs. It is intended to achieve the patient's spiritual well-being, help patients remain optimistic during treatment, and help patients accept their new situation with post-stroke UI, maintain hope, increase motivation, and encourage patients to struggle through post-stroke challenges.

Emotional factors also affect the recovery of stroke patients, even patients who are have considered functionally independent at three months after stroke still experience social isolation, difficulty social participation, and depression [35]. Early adaptation can predict depressive symptoms six months after stroke [35]. Emotional contro/emotional regulation is the process by which individuals influence the emotional that they have, when they have them, how they experience and express those emotions [49]. Emotional regulation is closely related to coping, emotional resilience, emotional intelligence, emotional expressiveness, and emotional energy.

In emotional control there are two strategies that are commonly used, namely reappraisal (reassessment) and suppression. Reappraisal occurs when the person changes the way he or she thinks about a potentially emotional situation and turn the experience into a non-emotional situation, whereas suppression is referred to as an obstacle to the way a person responds or behaves in an event that evokes emotion. In addition, social context also influences emotion regulation in various ways. Having attachment figures, friends, parents, spouse, children, and significant others are valuable interpersonal resources for dealing with emotions, expectations about their accessibility, assistance, and sensitivity can significantly increase or impair the capacity to manage emotions.

Based on this, the interventions/steps that need to be taken in controlling emotions include:

- Assess the patient's thought, feelings, and emotions.
- Show understanding, empathy, concern, and courtesy in communicating with patients.
- Help patients find and recognize the causes of emotions.
- Help patients to eliminate existing irrational thoughts through increasing knowledge about urinary incontinence.
- Assess the coping mechanisms used by the patient
- Advise and teach deep breathing relaxation techniques
- Involve the patient's family and people closest to the patient
- Instruct the family to avoid the patient from the environment or situation that can trigger the patient's emotions

5.4 Improving the ability to perform activities independently according to patient's ability

In Orem's theory (self-care deficit theory of nursing), Orem believes that human have the ability to care for themselves and if this ability is distorted, nurses help individuals to regain their abilities by providing direct care [32]. The results of our previous qualitative research showed that the informants' ability to carry out activities of daily living was in accordance with their ability to describe the conditions included in the supportive-educative system [36].

The supportive-educational system in Orem's theory states that individuals can do or can learn to take necessary actions externally or therapeutic self-care but cannot do so without help [28]. For this reason, guidance from nurses and caregivers are needed. However, in carrying out self-care activities emphasize the active role of patients in their health care rather than a passive role. It is necessary to make efforts to increase the self-care ability of post-stroke UI patients by involving patients in daily activities, but still being given supervision and help from caregivers in stages.

5.5 Improving family support and peer's attention

Social support can act as moderator of the effect of disability on well-being [35]. Support can be defined as help that a person can use in difficult situations. Support reduces the risk of mental and somatic disorders, modulates approaches to coping with stress, and reduces the likelihood of premature death [50, 51]. Social and emotional support is important for quality of life [51]. High levels of social support are associated with better mental health [52].

Family support and peer attention are often recommended as sources of emotional, instrumental, informational, and affirmative support for people with chronic disease conditions [22]. Family and peer support programs are an effective way to meet patient needs. Orem believes that the lack of social support to reassure patients in complex care situations leads to limitations in self-care behaviors [28].

Families contribute to maintaining the patient's well-being through emotional, instrumental, and practical support. Previous research has shown the effectiveness of treatment by involving the family in patient care [53]. However, in involving families as caregivers in patient care, it is necessary to be equipped with knowledge and skills related to patient care, caregivers must also be able to take care of their own health when caring for patients. The results of our previous qualitative study found that caregivers experience fatigue when caring for patients at home [36]. Fatigue and lack of rest experienced by caregivers are caused by the increased responsibility of caregivers in maintaining patient health [54]. Caregivers recognize that it is important to take care of their personal health so they can continue to care for their sick family members [54].

In addition to caregivers, peer attention is also needed. The results of qualitative study stated that informant felt very happy with the presence of a friend who also experienced the same disease as the informant, they shared their experiences during post-stroke UI [36]. Attention from peer who also experienced the same illness can help reduce feeling of isolation and fear, where peer support can be done by sharing experiences and providing information about the health services they need [22].

6. Model implementation guide

This model is implemented in five activities. The first activity was carried out at the hospital in the form of health education to patients and caregivers about post-stroke UI. The second activity is also carried out at the hospital and continued at the patient's home, in the form of skills training that needs to be given in the management of post-stroke UI including bladder retraining, pelvic floor muscle exercises, deep breathing exercises, ROM exercises, positive thinking exercises, and exercises controlling emotions. The third activity is in the form of assistance in implementing the skills that have been taught, this can be done at the patient's home. The fourth activity is in the form of monitoring and evaluation of patient's ability (patient independence), which can be done through home visits and telephone calls. The fifth activity is a follow-up. Follow-up can be done four weeks after all activities have been carried out.

7. Conclusion

Urinary incontinence is not only a physical problem, but also psychological and social problems. Post-stroke UI patients' still carry residual symptoms even through them have been discharged from the hospital. Management post-stroke UI in a holistic and continuous care manner up to the patient's home is needed to increase the patient's independent in overcoming the disease. Thus the achievement of the quality of life of post-stroke UI patients can be better.

Author details

Heltty Heltty[1,2]*, Ratna Sitorus[2], Nury Nusdwinuringtyas[3] and Evi Martha[4]

1 Lembaga Layanan Pendidikan Tinggi Wilayah IX Sulawesi, Indonesia

2 Department of Medical Surgical, Fakultas Ilmu Keperawatan, Universitas Indonesia, Depok, Indonesia

3 Department of Medic Rehabilitation, Fakultas Ilmu Kedokteran, Universitas Indonesia, Depok, Indonesia

4 Department of Public Health, Fakultas Ilmu Kesehatan Masyarakat, Universitas Indonesia, Depok, Indonesia

*Address all correspondence to: helttyheltty75@gmail.com; dindakeisha01@gmail.com

References

[1] Bizovicar N. Managing of lower urinary tract dysfunction following stroke. Current Bladder Dysfunction Report. 2018;13:125-131.DOI:10.1007/s11884-018-0472-5

[2] Arkan G, Beser A, Ozturk V. Experiences related to urinary incontinence of stroke patients: A qualitative descriptive study. Journal of Neuroscience Nursing. 2018;50(1):42-47. DOI:10.1097/JNN.0000000000000336

[3] Turhan N, Atalay A, Atabel HK. Impact of stroke etiology, lesion location and aging on post-stroke urinary incontinence as a predictor of functional recovery. International Journal of Rehabilitation Research. 2006;29:335-338. DOI: 10.1097/MRR.0b013e328010c7d1

[4] Junqueira J, Santos V. Urinary incontinence in hospital patients: Prevalence and associated factors. Revista Latino-Americana de Enfermagem. 2020;25:1-8. DOI: 10.1590/1518-8345.2139.2970

[5] Di M, Giovanni R. The impact of incontinence management on informal caregivers' quality of life. Aging Clinical and Experiment Research. 2015. DOI: 10.1007/s40520-015-0367-7

[6] Gotoh M. Matsukawa Y, Yoshikawa Y, Funahashi Y. Impact of urinary incontinence on the psychological burden of family caregivers. Neurology and Urodynamics. 2009;496(10):492-496. DOI: 10.1002/nau.20675

[7] Ge TJ, Vetter J, Lai HH. Sleep disturbance and fatique are associated with more severe urinary incontinence and overactive bladder symptoms. Journal of Urology. 2017;109:67-73. DOI: 10.1016/j.jurology.2017.07.039

[8] Senra C, Pereira MG. Quality of life in women with urinary incontinence. Rev Assoc Med Brass. 2015;61(2):178-183. DOI: 10.1590/1806-9282.61.02.178

[9] Elbana HM, Salama AM, Barakat MM. Effect of urinary incontinence on quality of life and self-esteem of postmenopausal women. American Journal of nursing science. 2018;7(5):182-191. DOI: 10.11648/j.ajns.20180705.15

[10] Mehdi Z, Birns J, Bhalla A. Post-stroke urinary incontinence. The International of Clinica Practice. 2013;67(11):1128-1137. DOI: 10.1111/ijcp.12183

[11] Heymen S. Psychological and cognitive variables affecting treatment outcomes for urinary and fecal incontinence. Journal of Gastroenterological. 2004:146-151. DOI: 10.1053/j.gastro.2003.10.040

[12] Chou YC, Jiang YH, Harnod T, Lee HT, Kuo HC. Stroke and lower urinary tract symptoms: A neurosurgical view. Urological Science. 2019;30(1):40-41. DOI: 10.4103/UROS.UROS_82_18

[13] Matthews M, Mitchell EA. Causes and rehabilitation of urinary incontinence after stroke: A literature review. Nursing and Residential Care. 2010;12(10):474-481. DOI: 10.12968/nrec.2010.12.10.78403

[14] Jamieson K, Brady M, Peacock C. Urinary dysfunction: Assessment and management in stroke patients. Nursing Standard. 2010;25(3):49-55. DOI: 10.7748/ns2010.09.25.3.49.c7991

[15] Dumoulin C, Komer-betensky N, Tannenbaum C. Identification, Assessment, and Intervention by rehabilitation professionals in Canada. Journal of The American Heart Association. 2007. DOI: 10.1161/STROKEAHA.107.486035

[16] Thomas LH, Coupe J, Cross LD, Tan AL, Watkins CL. Interventions for treating urinary incontinence after stroke in adults (Review). Cochrane Database of Systematic Reviews. 2019. DOI: 10.1002/14651858.CD004462.pub4.

[17] Rizvi RM, Ather MH. Assessment of urinary incontinence (UI) in adult patients. IntechOpen. 2017. DOI: 10.5772/66953

[18] Sharaf AY, Sebai NA, Ewieda SM, Shokry MS, Salem MA. The impact of nursing interventions on the control of urinary incontinence among women. Journal of America Science. 2010;6(10): 1256-1271. ISSN: 1545-1003

[19] French B, Thomas LH, Harrison J, Coupe J, Roe B, Booth J, et al. Client and clinical staff perceptions of barriers to and enablers of the uptake and delivery of behavioral interventions for urinary incontinence: Qualitative evidence synthesis. The Journal of Advanced Nursing. 2016:1-18. DOI: 10.1111/jan.13083

[20] Burgio KL. Behavioral treatment options for urinary incontinence. American Gastroenterological Association. 2004;126:82-89. DOI: 10.1053/j.gastro.2003.10.042

[21] Kneebone II. A framework to support cognitive behavior therapy for emotional disorder after stroke. Cognitive and Behavioral Practice. 2016;23:99-109. DOI: 10.1016/j.cbpra.2015.02.001

[22] Kessler D, Egan M, Kubina L. Peer support for stroke survivors: A case study. Biomed Central Health Service Research. 2014;14(1):1-9. DOI: 10.1186/1472-6963-14-256

[23] Garley A, Unwin JA. A case series to pilot cognitive behavior therapy for women with urinary incontinence. British Journal of Health Psychology. 2006;11:373-386. DOI: 10.1348/135910705X53876

[24] Griffiths D, Tadic SD. Bladder control, urgency, and urge incontinence: Evidence from functional bran imaging. Neurology and Urodynamics. 2008;474(2007):466-474. DOI: 10.1002/nau.20549

[25] Hassan GA, Ibrahim HS. The effect of supportive nursing intervention on burden and coping strategies of caregivers of children with cancer. Journal of Nursing Education and Practice. 2018;8(7):125-136. DOI: 10.5430/jnep.v8n7p125.

[26] Robb SL, Hanson-Abromeit D. A review of supportive care interventions to manage distress in young children with cancer and parent. Cancer Nursing Lippincott Williams & Wilkins. 2014;37(4). DOI: 10.1097/NCC.0000000000000095

[27] Navidian A, Ebrahimi H, Keykha R. Supportive nursing care and satisfaction of patients receiving electroconvulsive therapy: A randomized controlled clinical trial. Iran Red Crescent Med Journal. 2015;17(9):e27492. DOI: 10.5812/ircmj.27492

[28] Alligood MR. Nursing theory: Utilization and application. 5th ed. Elsevier Mosby; 2014

[29] Hansen-Ketchum P. Parse's theory in practice an interpretive analysis. Journal of Holistic Nursing. 2004;22(1): 57-72. DOI: 10.1177/0898010103261120

[30] Romeo JH. Comprehensive versus holistic care case studies of chronic disease. Journal of holistis nursing. 2000;18(4):352-361. DOI:10.1177/089801010001800406

[31] Wiwanitkit V. Cultural and spiritual dimension of chronic disease: an important concern for practitioners. International Journal of chronic diseases

and therapy. 2015;18(2014):7613. DOI: 10.19070/2572-7613-

[32] Wilson J, Gramling L. The application of Orem's Self-care Model. Research gate. 2017. DOI: 10.1097/BCR.0b013e3181b48a2d

[33] Arkan G, Beser A, Ozturk V, Bozkurt O, Gulbahar S. Effects on urinary outcome of patients and caregivers' burden of pelvic floor muscle exercises based on the health belief model done at home by post-stroke patients. Topics in Stroke Rehabilitation. 2018. DOI: 10.1080/10749357.2018.1552741

[34] Dumoulin C, Korner-Bitensky N, Tannenbaum C. Urinary incontinence after stroke: Does rehabilitation make a difference? A systematic review of the effectiveness of behavioral therapy. Pubmed. 2005;12(3):66-67. DOI: 10.1310/ENMX-RUV5-15WL-VNA2

[35] Artal FJC, Egido JA. Quality of life after stroke: The important of a good recovery. Pubmed. 2009; 1(suppl1):204-14. DOI: 10.1159/000200461

[36] Heltty H, Sitorus R, Martha E, Nusdwinuringtyas N. Experience of the patient's success in faced a post-stroke urinary incontinence: The patient's perspective. Frontier of Nursing. 2021;8(3).

[37] Christalle E, Zill JM, Frerichs W, Harter M, Nestoriuc Y, Dirmaler J, et al. Assessment of patient information needs: A systematic review of measures. Plos One. 2019;14(1). DOI: 10.1371/journal.pone.0209165

[38] Kelley T, Docherty S, Brandon D. Information needed to support knowing the patient. Advances in Nursing Science. 2014;36(4):351-363. DOI: 10.1097/ANS.0000000000000000.6

[39] Hunter KF, Wagg AS. Improving nurse engagement in continence care. Nursing Research and reviews. 2018. DOI: 10.2147/NRR.S144356

[40] Mata KR, Costa RC, Carbone ED, Gimenez MM, Bortolini MA, Castro RA, et al. Telehealth in the rehabilitation of female pelvic floor dysfunction: A systematic literature review. International Urogynecology Journal. 2021;32:249-259. DOI: 10.1007/s00192-020-04588-8

[41] Bournes DA, Naef R. Human becoming practice around the globe: Exploring the art of living true presence. Nursing Science Quarterly. 2006;19(2):109-115. DOI: 10.1177/089431840628632

[42] Bahrami S, Heidari M, Hamta A, Samadi F, Heida A. Relationship of religious attitude and self-control with quality of life among student of university of QOM and QOM university of medical science: A path analysis. Health, Spiritual and Medical Ethics. 2019. DOI: 10.29252/jhsme.6.2.2

[43] Araujo G, Lins I, Armendaris MK, Lucia D, Pinho M, Kamada I, et al. Theory of human becoming in nursing ecology: Applying Meleis' evaluation method. Text Context Nursing. Florianopolis. 2013;22(4):1179-1186. DOI: 10.1590/S0104-170720130 00400037

[44] Mousavi E, Esmaeili A, Saless SS. The effect of positive thinking on quality of life and resiliency of cancer patients. Razavi International Journal of Medicine. 2015;3(3). DOI: 10.17795/rijm27122

[45] Elfatah WA. The effectiveness of self-control and anxiety management training to reduce anxiety and improve health-related quality of life in children with asthma. Journal of Psychology & Psychotherapy. 2015. DOI: 10.4172/2161-0487.1000220

[46] Kirkegaard-Weston E. Positive thinking: Toward a conceptual model

and organizational implication. Pace University. 2005.

[47] Naseem Z, Khalid R. Positive thinking in coping with stress and health outcomes: Literature review. Journal of Research and Reflection in Education. 2010;4(1):42-61. http://www.ue.edu.pk/jrre

[48] Laurin K, Kay AC, Fitzsimons M. Divergent effects of activating thoughts of God on self-regulation. Journal of Personality and Social Psychology. 2012;102:4-21. DOI: 10.1037/a0025971

[49] Fasbinder A, Shidler K, Caboral-Stevens M. A concept analysis: Emotional regulation of nurses. Nursing Forum Wiley. 2019. DOI: 10.1111/nuf.12405

[50] Zdun-Ry'zewskaa A, Basi'nskia K, Majkowicza M, Podolskab M, Landowskic J, Walden-Galuszko K. Association between social support and quality of life in patients with affective disorders. The European Journal of Psychiatry. 2018. DOI: 10.1016/j.ejpsy.2018.05.002

[51] Kobayashi R, Ishizaki M. Relationship between health literacy and social support and the quality of lif in patients with cancer: Questionnaire study. Journal of Participatory Medicine. 2020;12(1):e17163. DOI: 10.2196/17163

[52] Bosworth, H., Siegler, I., Olsen, M., Brummett, B., Barefoot, J., Williams, R., et al. Social support and quality of life in patients with coronary artery disease. Quality of Life Research. 2000;9(7):829-39. DOI: 10.1023/a:1008960308011

[53] Plant H, Moore S, Richardson A, Cornwall A, Medina J, Ream E. Nurses' experience of delivering a supportive intervention for family members of patients with lung cancer. European Journal of Cancer Care. 2011;20:436-444. DOI: 10.1111/j.1365-2354.2011.01249.

[54] Maciasaac BL, Harrison MB, Buchanan D, Hopman WM. Supportive care needs after an acute stroke: A descriptive enquiry of careivers' perspective. Journal of Neuroscience Nursing. 2011;43(3):132-40. DOI: 10.1097/JNN.0b013e3182135b28.

Chapter 7

Rehabilitation Protocols for Children with Dysfunctional Voiding

Vesna D. Zivkovic, Ivona Stankovic, Lidija Dimitrijevic, Hristina Colovic, Dragan Zlatanovic and Natasa Savic

Abstract

Dysfunctional voiding is a functional voiding disorder characterized by an intermittent uroflow rate due to involuntary intermittent contractions of the striated muscle of the external urethral sphincter or pelvic floor muscles (PFMs) during voiding in neurologically normal children. Symptoms include voiding difficulties as well as urgency, voiding frequency and, in some instances, urinary incontinence and/or nocturnal enuresis. Recurrent urinary tract infections, chronic constipation and/or fecal incontinence and vesicoureteral reflux (VUR) contribute to this condition. Urotherapy is the mainstay of the treatment. It starts with education and demystification and simple behavioral modifications. Specific measures include PFM exercises with various forms of biofeedback concentrating at the recognition of PFM function and their relaxation. However, the PFMs are part of the abdominal capsule and they act in coordination with lower abdominal muscles. These muscles need to be relaxed during voiding. Diaphragmatic breathing exercises were introduced to teach children abdominal muscle relaxation. Easy to learn exercises do not require any specific equipment and can be performed at all health care levels. Children from five years of age could benefit from these exercises.
In children resistant to standard treatment, botulinum toxin type A application, intermittent catheterization and surgery in children with VUR are recommended.

Keywords: dysfunctional voiding, urotherapy, pelvic floor exercises, diaphragmatic breathing exercises, pelvic floor electromyography biofeedback

1. Introduction

Disorders of bladder and bowel control are among the most common problems in childhood. At the age of 7, 10% of children get wet during the night, 2 to 3% wet their clothes during the day, while 1 to 3% of children have fecal incontinence [1]. These disorders often occur together. Despite a high rate of spontaneous remission, 1 to 2% of adolescents have nocturnal enuresis and less than 1% have daily urinary incontinence or fecal incontinence [2]. Most of these disorders are functional, i.e. they are not caused by neurological, structural, or medical factors.

Functional voiding disorders are some of the main causes of daily wetting in children, the development of recurrent urinary tract infections and vesicoureteral reflux (VUR). In addition to the risk of developing structural changes in the bladder wall and upper urinary tract, voiding disorders, accompanied by urinary incontinence, can be a severe psychosocial problem. Children describe wetting at school as the third most stressful event in life after the death of a parent and loss of sight [3]. It is evident that urinary incontinence causes significant psychological morbidity, and treatment is crucial.

Functional voiding disorders can be treated in a number of ways, including pharmacological therapy, urotherapy, and surgical treatment in the most severe cases.

2. Dysfunctional voiding

2.1 Definition

Dysfunctional voiding (DV) refers only to the disorder of the bladder emptying phase, and is characterized by intermittent contraction of the external urethral sphincter and/or PFMs during the voiding phase of a micturition cycle [4]. A typical finding is interuppted or staccato uroflowmetry curve with increased electromyography (EMG) pelvic floor muscle activity during urination.

The more severe form is referred to as Hinman syndrome by the author who first described it [5]. Other terms previously used for DV are detrusor-sphincter discoordination, non-neurogenic neurogenic bladder and occult neurogenic bladder. In the United States, the term "dysfunctional voiding" has been used for all types of voiding disorders, even bladder filling phase disorders. According to the ICCS standardization of terminology from 2016, DV refers exclusively to the disorder of the voiding phase [4]. It is thought to be the result of excessive PFM activity in an attempt to prevent urination that occurs due to uninhibited detrusor contractions in the early stage of bladder filling.

2.2 Epidemiology

Epidemiological data on DV are lacking. Dysfunctional voiding was found to occur in 4.2% of children referred for urinary incontinence [6]. In published studies, the prevalence was estimated to be between 5 and 25% and 32% [7, 8]. Dysfunctional voiding was observed in 65% of children aged 5-9 years with urinary tract infections, and in 23% of children who were urinary tract infections free [9]. It is evident that the criteria for including children in the studies were different, as well as the accuracy of their evaluation, which indicates the need to conduct new research to determine accurate data.

2.3 Etiology

Dysfunctional voiding was first observed in 1973 by Hinman and Baumann [5]. Hinman describes it as an acquired, reversible behavioral disorder that can be ameliorated by suggestion and changes in behavior. He defined it as a bad habit for special people in a bad family environment. Allen stated in 1977 that hyperactivity of a child is a typical sign and that psychological factors play a key role in at least 50% of the 21 children described [10]. He also points to the importance of stressful situations in the family, such as parental alcoholism, parental divorce and father dominance.

Contrary to these considerations, Van Gool points out that DV is not related to emotional or psychosocial problems, but is caused by delayed CNS maturation and external urethral sphincter dysfunction [11]. Hjalmas considers the importance of hereditary factors, as DV was observed in several members of the same family [12]. It is not known whether this is due to genetic factors or common family habits.

Most authors, however, believe that DV is a learned behavior [13]. It can develop from overactive bladder (OAB) and voiding postponement as a result of PFM contractions in an attempt to prevent urination, but it can also exist without these precursors. In some children, urgency, voiding frequency and, in some instances, urinary incontinence and signs of DV are present at the same time [14].

From the review of the literature so far, it can be concluded that the etiology is probably multifactorial. Possible risk factors are:

1. Inadequate toilet training process

   Wiener et al. suggest that functional voiding disorders may be caused by inadequate toilet habits and postures [15], which was also confirmed in the study by Bakker et al. [16]. This study indicated that the use of adult toilets in the process of children's toilet training may increase the risk of developing functional voiding disorders. Thus, most of the programmes used in the treatment of DV involve taking an adequate position when urinating, i.e. the use of a toilet insert and footrests to ensure the stability of the trunk and the relaxation of the PFMs, and thus enable the physiological emptying of the bladder.

2. Small structural anomalies in the anatomy or innervation of the lower urinary tract.

3. Delay in maturation: detrusor overactivity as a component of DV may represent the persistence of normal infantile mode of urination even after toilet training. It is possible that delays in CNS maturation reduce the ability of these children to take voluntary control of the micturition reflex.

4. Impact of school: more than half of the time children spend in school, which suggests that teachers can positively or negatively influence the acquisition of toilet habits. In a study by Cooper et al., the influence of schools on the development of DV in children was examined and it was pointed out that most teachers allow going to the toilet only during rest [17]. Such a ban on going to the toilet for a child with an urgency who has not yet developed a complete inhibition of the micturition reflex may impair the normal function of the urinary bladder and sphincter. In addition, most children with daily urinary incontinence avoided going to the school toilet due to lack of privacy or poor toilet hygiene [17].

5. Unpleasant events during toilet training and/or personal stress: serious emotional stresses, such as sexual abuse, mostly of girls, should be considered in the event of sudden onset of DV, and in the absence of other etiological factors [18].

2.4 Clinical signs and symptoms

Children are usually referred for wetting clothes, but not for DV. Children and parents usually do not register specific symptoms of DV, so the physician must insist on them. Typical signs are difficulty initiating micturition (hesitancy), as well as straining to overcome the resistance of the contracted urinary sphincter. The urinary stream is usually not strong because the PFMs do not relax completely, and it is often intermittent.

In an attempt to postpone voiding or suppress urgency and/or urinary incontinence, children assume characteristic positions such as crossing their legs, standing on tiptoes, squatting, or manual compression of the genitals (pelvic holding maneuvers). It is typical for girls to squat by pressing their heel against the perineum [19].

Stool retention, chronic constipation and fecal incontinence occur in more than 50% of children as a result of repeated and habitual contractions of the PFMs [9].

Plenty of data from the literature indicate an association between DV and recurrent urinary tract infections [8, 20–22]. Treatment of DV reduces recurrent urinary tract infections. About 50% of children with DV may have VUR [10].

2.5 Hinman-Allen syndrome

The most severe form of DV is Hinman-Allen syndrome, according to the authors who first described it in 1973 [5, 10]. The old term "non-neurogenic neurogenic bladder" can also be found in the literature.

This syndrome occurs in children who voluntarily and habitually contract the external urethral sphincter during uninhibited detrusor contractions, which leads to the inability of emptying the bladder. The condition is characterized by detrusor overactivity and possibly its decompensation. It is clinically manifested by daytime and nighttime wetting, urgency and overflow incontinence, chronic constipation, as well as recurrent urinary tract infections. Voiding cystourethrography reveals a trabeculated bladder, high-grade bilateral VUR and large post-void residual urine. If not treated in time, it leads to reflux nephropathy followed by kidney scarring, hypertension and progressive renal failure.

3. Evaluation of a child with dysfunctional voiding

Evaluation of children with DV includes taking anamnestic data, physical examination, filling in the bladder and bowel diary, urinalyses and urine culture, ultrasound examination of the bladder and kidneys and uroflowmetry with determination of post-void residual urine. Cystometry, voiding cystourethrography and MRI of the spine are indicated only in certain cases.

3.1 History

The evaluation process begins with anamnesis, data on perinatal factors, developmental course, current mental state, school success and events during toilet training. Every child should be asked how he urinates, whether he has difficulty starting to urinate, whether urinating is difficult and whether he strains when urinating. Also, one should insist on the characteristics of the urinary stream, such as strength and continuity. A weak and intermittent stream indicates the existence of DV. The child should be asked if he has a feeling of incomplete urination or urinary retention (inability to urinate). Questions regarding urgency, voiding frequency and severity of daytime and nighttime wetting, pelvic holding maneuvers, and bowel emptying should follow.

3.2 Physical examination

3.2.1 Abdominal examination

Palpation of the left iliac fossa is necessary in order to determine fecal impaction. Suprapubic tenderness may indicate the presence of cystitis. If urine leaks when the bladder is pressed, the existence of a neurogenic bladder with sphincter damage should be suspected.

3.2.2 Neurological examination

It is necessary to perform a careful inspection of the lower part of the spine in order to determine the cutaneous manifestations of occult spinal dysraphism and/or sacral agenesis (lipomas, nevi, increased hairiness, low intergluteal cleft, flattened buttocks). After that, it is necessary to test the tendon reflexes on the lower extremities as well as the existence of the Babinski sign. Hyperreflexia, asymmetry in reflexes or positive Babinski indicate spinal cord damage. It is also important to examine the strength of the muscles of the lower extremities, ataxia and gait.

3.2.3 Inspection of genitals and perianal region

Genital inspection is necessary in every patient with DV. Inspection of the perineum reveals the position of the anus, fissure, fistula or perianal inflammation of the skin in children with constipation.

3.2.4 Rectal examination

Digital rectal examination can determine the tone and function of the anal sphincter, the width and content of the rectal ampulla, the amount and consistency of feces in the ampulla, and the presence of pain. It is recommended that anorectal examination be performed only in those children who meet 1 of 6 Rome III criteria for the diagnosis of constipation [9].

3.3 Bladder and bowel diary

The bladder diary is a crucial diagnostic and therapeutic instrument for children with voiding disorders. After the anamnesis and physical examination, this is the third most important part of the evaluation. It is used to understand and quantify the function of the bladder at home, because the memory of the elements of voiding is unreliable. A complete bladder diary is kept for 7 nights and urinary incontinence is registered, as well as nocturnal urine volume, in order to evaluate nocturnal enuresis [4].

The 48 hr. daytime frequency and volume chart is kept for 48 hours, preferably on weekends for practical reasons [4]. The data obtained are frequency of voiding, volume of individual urination, maximum voided volume, urine production, nocturia, nocturnal urine production and fluid intake. The frequency of voiding in children with DV is variable.

A bowel diary is kept for 7 days to rule out the presence of constipation [4]. The frequency of defecation, the appearance of the stool according to the Bristol scale, pain and tension during defecation, whether the child has previously delayed defecation and whether fecal incontinence is present are entered.

3.4 Urinalysis and urine culture

Urinalyses and urine culture are initial tests to rule out urinary tract infection.

3.5 Urodynamics

3.5.1 Uroflowmetry

Uroflowmetry is the simplest form of urodynamics. As a non-invasive method, it is ideal for pediatric needs (**Figure 1**). It enables the examination of the function of the detrusor and the sphincter in the voiding phase of the child's micturition.

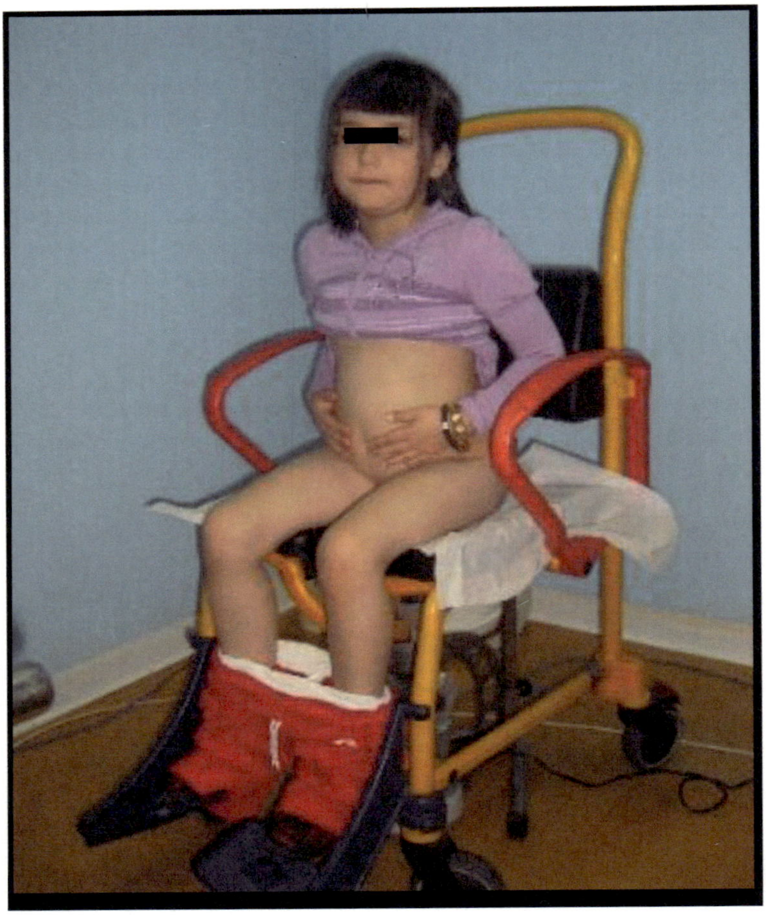

Figure 1.
Uroflowmetry.

The uroflowmeter was first described in the 1950s [23]. The method can be applied from the fourth year of life of a child with established micturition control. In order to get reliable results, it is necessary for the child to urinate at a capacity that is not less than 50% nor more than 115% of the bladder capacity expected for age [4]. In addition, it is necessary to repeat examination to make the result accurate and reliable.

The method consists in urinating the patient in a uroflowmeter, continuously measuring the urine flow rate (ml/s) and at the same time graphically showing the curve. The placement of two superficial EMG electrodes on the perineum enables the recording of the activity of the PFMs in the micturition phase. In this way, significant data are obtained, especially in children with DV. The uroflowmetry curve is of the staccato or interrupted type with an increase in the EMG activity of the PFMs during urination (**Figure 2**).

Upon completion of this study, an ultrasound examination of the bladder is performed to determine post-void residual urine. In a child aged 7 to 12 years, residual urine greater than 20 ml or 15% of the bladder capacity expected for age is considered elevated [4]. Residual urine that is larger than 10 ml or 6% of bladder capacity expected for age during several measurements is also considered elevated [4].

3.5.2 Cystometry

Cystometry is the only method by which bladder function can be examined directly and in detail. The method is invasive. In order to obtain the data necessary

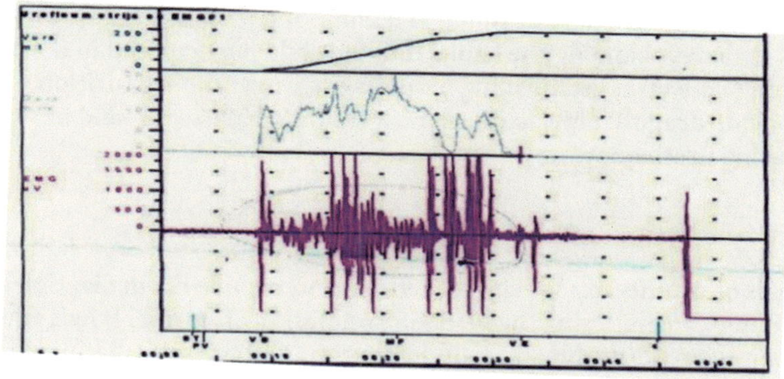

Figure 2.
Interrupted uroflowmetry curve with increased pelvic floor EMG activity during voiding.

for urodynamic analysis of bladder function, simultaneous measurement of pressure in the bladder, urethra and abdomen is required. This continuous measurement of detrusor pressure and sphincter activity during bladder filling and emptying allows an accurate diagnosis to be made for most lower urinary tract disorders.

In children with DV, cystometry is indicated only in certain cases, primarily because the diagnosis is made using non-invasive methods. It should be performed only in severe cases of DV, which should be differentially and diagnostically distinguished from neurogenic bladder with detrusor sphincter dyssynergia, suspicion of Hinman-Allen syndrome and DV resistant to the applied therapy.

3.6 Voiding cystourethrography (VCUG)

Voiding cystourethrography is not routinely performed in children with DV. It is used in children with recurrent urinary tract infections to rule out the presence of VUR. A typical finding in DV is a ballooned proximal urethra. If ultrasound examination reveals bladder wall thickening and hydronephrosis and/or a plateau uroflowmetry curve, it is necessary to perform VCUG to exclude the presence of a posterior urethral valve in boys.

3.7 Magnetic resonance imaging

Magnetic resonance imaging (MRI) of the spine should be performed in every child with a suspected neurogenic voiding disorder or in whom a clinical examination has established the existence of spinal dysraphism. Suspicion of tethered cord syndrome, as well as spinal tumors, are also indications for referring a child for an MRI of the spine.

4. Urotherapy

Functional voiding disorders should be actively treated due to the possibility of developing structural changes in the bladder and upper urinary tract. In the Anglo-Saxon literature, the term "urotherapy" has been used since 1980 in children with voiding disorders, which is synonymous with rehabilitation of the lower urinary tract [24].

4.1 Definition

Urotherapy is a conservative, non-surgical treatment of the lower urinary tract and can be defined as re-education of the bladder or rehabilitation programme aimed at correcting the phase of filling and emptying the bladder [4]. Urotherapy, first of all, includes changing the habits that the child has acquired in the process of toilet training, as well as establishing motor control over the micturition reflex. It can also include drug therapy, because most children have some kind of pharmacotherapy during urotherapy.

4.2 Goals

The goals of urotherapy are clearly defined and include normalization of the phase of filling and emptying the bladder, facilitation of normal bowel function and normalization of the dynamics of defecation. The goals of treatment in clinical practice are aimed at reducing urgency and urinary incontinence, nocturnal enuresis, post-void residual urine, high intravesical pressure, PFM activity in the micturition phase, normalization of uroflowmetry curve, cure urinary tract infections and constipation, and reduce the degree of VUR.

4.3 Indications

Urotherapy is used in functional voiding disorders that are accompanied by an altered phase of bladder filling and emptying, in children in whom satisfactory results have not been achieved with the use of pharmacological therapy, and in children who are just starting therapy.

4.4 Components of urotherapy

Urotherapy consists of standard urotherapy and specific measures that include neuromodulation, PFM relaxation exercises, biofeedback and intermittent catheterization [4].

4.4.1 Standard urotherapy

In the literature, we often come across the term "standard urotherapy", which includes education, behavioral modifications, keeping a bladder and bowel diary and regular check-ups [4]. Before starting urotherapy, it is necessary to dedicate a lot of time to educating the child, examining his motivation to carry out the treatment, and eliminating the shame and other effects that urinary incontinence can cause.

4.4.1.1 Education and demystification

The child should be acquainted with the structure and function of the bladder, external urinary sphincter, colon and anorectum in a way that is appropriate for his age. He also needs to be explained the etiology of his voiding and defecation disorders. It is important to examine the motivation for treatment. If the child is not motivated, the results of the treatment are much worse.

4.4.1.2 Behavioral modifications

The goal is to improve the control of urination and defecation through changes in the child's behavior. This includes regular voiding and hydration, taking the correct position during urination and defecation, as well as changing the diet. With the application of this initial treatment, a cure can be achieved in about 20% of children [21].

4.4.1.3 Regular hydration

Children with voiding disorders are often voluntarily dehydrated. Concentrated urine can cause irritation and burning when urinating. The introduction of adequate hydration (200 ml 5-6 times a day) increases urine production and bladder capacity, reduces urine concentration and improves bowel function. It is forbidden to drink beverages such as Coca-Cola, coffee, tea, cold juices, because they can induce detrusor overactivity [25].

4.4.1.4 Regular voiding

It is the basis of bladder rehabilitation and includes the adoption of a voiding schedule every 2-3 hours. The goal is to prevent bladder distension, to restore the feeling of fullness of the bladder, and to reduce the hyperactivity of the bladder. The child and parents should know that the ability to start micturition, even when the child does not want to urinate, is an important step in controlling the continence and emptying of the bladder. The child should try to urinate only at a predetermined time, and avoid delaying urination. It is necessary to analyze the child's daily activities and determine the time of micturition accordingly.

4.4.1.5 Optimal bladder emptying

The position when urinating has a significant effect on the ability to empty the bladder. Toilet bowls are intended for adults and as such are not suitable for children. Relaxation of the PFMs is difficult or impossible with various irregular positions that the child assumes during urination.

Proper voiding position means urinating in a sitting position on the toilet bowl for girls and boys. For smaller children, it is important to require the use of an adequate toilet seat insert and footrests to ensure trunk stability [26]. When urinating, the child should be slightly bent forward, with the spine in extension, the hips in abduction and the relaxed abdominal muscles (**Figure 3**). It is necessary for children to listen to the sound of the stream when urinating and the goal is for the stream to be strong, long and sonorous.

4.4.1.6 Treatment of chronic constipation/fecal incontinence

It is important to recognize the defecation disorder, because it has been proven that the treatment of constipation alone significantly reduces the symptoms of the lower urinary tract. In the group of children with increased post-void residual urine and constipation, 66% had an improvement in bladder emptying after constipation treatment. Urinary incontinence, nocturnal enuresis, and recurrent urinary tract infections were cured in most children treated only for constipation [20]. Therefore, treatment begins with chronic constipation management.

In the treatment of chronic constipation, four steps are applied: education, disimpaction of fecal mass, prevention of its re-accumulation and follow-up [27]. Treatment is usually applied for 3-6 months, but the relapses are frequent [28]. The cure rate of chronic functional constipation after application of standard treatment that includes laxatives and behavioral approaches is only 50-60% [29].

More than half of children with chronic constipation have an abnormal defecation pattern because they contract the external anal sphincter and the *M. puborectalis* during defecation [30]. This form of abnormal defecation is considered to be learned resulting from the habit of delaying defecations. Physiotherapy

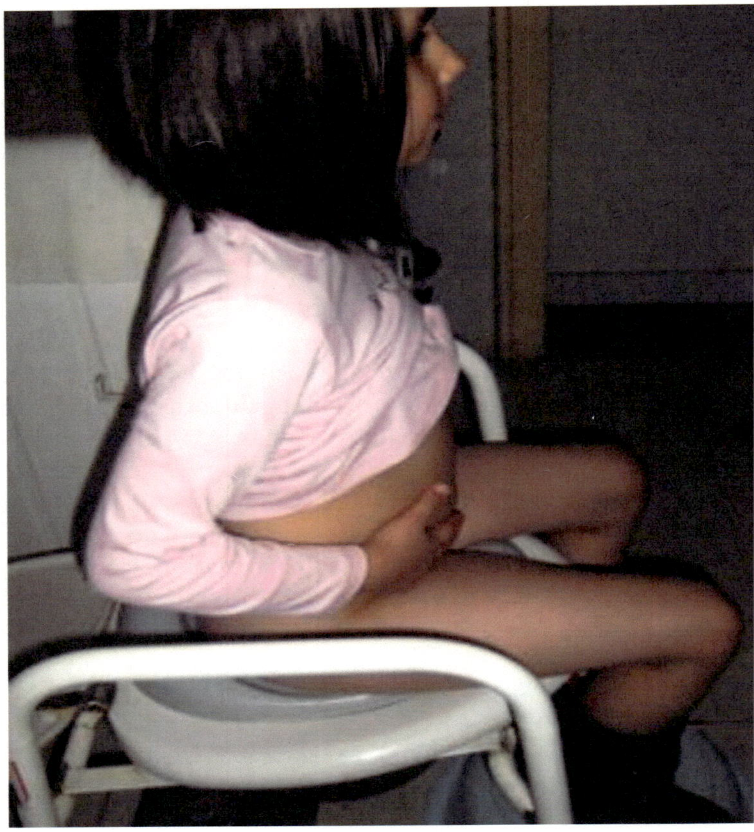

Figure 3.
Correct position when urinating.

interventions such are diaphragmatic breathing exercises and pelvic floor exercises with or without biofeedback were introduced in order to educate a child to relax the external anal sphincter and the PFMs during defecation [31–35]. In refractory cases, even botulinum toxin injections are administrated into the external anal sphincter [36].

Interferential current stimulation (IFS) has been used in the treatment of chronic constipation resistant to standard therapy in children. Significant improvements in clinical symptoms (increased frequency of defecation, reduction of fecal incontinence and abdominal pain) were seen in 67% of children and lasted for more than two years in one third of the treated patients [37]. In addition, the time of colonic transit on colonic scintigraphy was shorter after the application of IFS [38]. Although the mechanism of action of IFS is still insufficiently known, the proposed theories are the activation of local sensory nerves in the skin, spinal nerves (sensory and motor T9-L2), sympathetic and parasympathetic nerves in the intestine, enteric nerves, pacemaker cells (Cajal's interstitial cells) or smooth muscle cells in the intestinal wall [39].

5. Rehabilitation protocols for dysfunctional voiding

Although there is no general approach to treatment and treatment varies from one patient to another, there are several ways to treat children with DV, including urotherapy, pharmacotherapy, botulinum toxin application, and surgical treatment in children with VUR.

In addition to standard urotherapy, special measures are applied, such as exercises for relaxation of PFMs with or without biofeedback and exercises for relaxation of abdominal muscles.

5.1 Pelvic floor muscle relaxation exercises and biofeedback

Pelvic floor muscle exercises were first used in pediatric urology by Wennergren and Oberg, with the aim of developing the child's awareness of their function [40]. During the exercises, the child learns to contract and relax these muscles without activating auxiliary muscles (gluteal and hip adductors). In order to improve voluntary control, the exercises can be combined with different types of biofeedback, such as visual (observation of the abdomen in front of a mirror), tactile (palpation of the PFMs or *M. transversus abdominis*), uroflowmetry or electromyography.

Biofeedback was first used by Maizels et al. in 1979, who implemented the use of urodynamics devices in children with detrusor sphincter dyssynergia [41]. During urination, children observed EMG activity of the sphincter. Improvement was achieved in two of the three treated children.

Uroflowmetry biofeedback consists of the child observing the uroflowmetry curve while urinating. During voiding, the child is advised to make sure that the curve is bell-shaped. Kjolseth examined the efficacy of uroflowmetry biofeedback in 32 children with DV [42]. The number of applied sessions was 1-9, while 47% of children required 4-5 sessions. Cure was achieved in 50% of children, improvement in 8 children, and 7 children were unchanged. The uroflowmetry curve was completely normalized in 55% of children. It has been shown that this type of biofeedback requires a smaller number of sessions compared to EMG biofeedback and leads to faster normalization of the act of urination [43].

5.1.1 Animated pelvic floor EMG biofeedback

Mc Kenna et al. in 1999 applied biofeedback in the form of interactive computer games that enabled the active participation of patients [44]. Computer play maintained the child's interest and motivation for the exercise programme. The method consists of placing superficial EMG electrodes on the child's perineum, and then the child is taught to properly contract and relax the PFMs by watching a game on a computer monitor. In this way, children become aware of the activity of the PFMs and learn to control them by controlling the activities of their favorite heroes (dolphin, monkey, fish, bee).

In a study by Herndon et al. interactive computer games were used in 160 children with DV [45]. In 87% of patients, subjective improvement of symptoms was achieved. In a study by McKenna et al. improvement of nocturnal enuresis was achieved in 90%, daily wetting in 89%, constipation and fecal incontinence in 100% [44].

Kaye and Palmer did not find significant differences in efficacy after application of non-animated (biofeedback without animation using only EMG tracing) and animated biofeedback [46]. However, a group of children who had animated biofeedback required a smaller number of sessions to normalize the uroflowmetry curve and reduce residual urine. In a study by Desantis et al. there was an improvement in urinary tract infections in 83%, diurnal incontinence in 80%, constipation from 18–100%, urinary frequency from 67–100%, urgency from 71–88% and VUR from 21–100% of children [47].

In a study by Palmer et al. in children with DV and VUR, the use of biofeedback accelerated the resolution of VUR or reduced the degree of VUR in 71% of children [48]. Similar results were presented by Khen-Dunlop et al. and Kibar et al. [49, 50].

Adequate patient selection seems to be the most important for biofeedback success. Parents and children should be motivated and compliant to continue practicing exercises at home [51].

Although numerous studies highlight the positive effects of PFM relaxation exercises with or without biofeedback, there is no clear recommendation of an exercise protocol to use in the rehabilitation of children with DV. The number of sessions, the number of repetitions, the duration of the contraction and relaxation phase, as well as the period of performing the exercises differ significantly between the studies.

De Paepe et al. applied PFM relaxation exercises with EMG biofeedback [52]. The protocol consisted of 30 submaximal contractions lasting 3 seconds, followed by a relaxation phase of 30 seconds. One session per week was applied for 6 months (maximum 20-24 sessions). In a study by Vasconcelos et al., 24 home exercise sessions lasting 20 minutes were applied, three times a week during a three-month period [53]. The contractions lasted for 5 seconds, followed by a 10-second relaxation period. Shei Dei increased the duration of contractions to 10 seconds and extended the relaxation period to 30 seconds [54]. Yagci et al. applied submaximal contractions of 3 seconds, followed by a relaxation period of 30 seconds [55]. The children repeated the exercises at home three times a day for 6 months. In a retrospective study, Drzeviecki et al. analyzed a programme in which the contractions lasted 10 seconds, followed by a relaxation of 10 seconds [56]. After that, fast contractions lasting 5 seconds and 5 seconds of relaxation followed. On average, 3 sessions (1-8) were applied.

5.2 Abdominal capsule

Sapsford et al. showed that the PFMs are not an isolated unit, but a part of the abdominal capsule that surrounds the abdominal and pelvic organs [57]. The structures that make this capsule are the lumbar vertebrae, *M. multifidus*, diaphragm, *M. transversus abdominis* and PFMs. These muscles contribute to maintaining the posture of the body in an upright position and act synergistically.

Coactivation of the abdominal and PFMs is necessary for the development of intra-abdominal pressure and contributes to the stability of the spine. It is shown that *M. transversus abdominis* contributes the most to the development of intra-abdominal pressure in relation to other abdominal muscles [58]. This muscle is first activated during functions related to the increase in intra-abdominal pressure, such as spinal stabilization and expiratory tasks [58]. Coactivation of the abdominal capsule muscles has been demonstrated during weight lifting, coughing and forced expiratory tasks [58, 59].

Pelvic floor muscle dysfunction can present as hyperactivity, leading to the development of voiding and defecation disorders, such as DV, chronic constipation, perianal and perineal pain. Many of these children have hyperactivity of the lower abdominal muscles, which do not relax during urination and defecation and thus prevent the relaxation of the PFMs [57].

5.3 Diaphragmatic breathing exercises

As lower abdominal muscles (*M. transversus abdominis* and *M. obliquus internus abdominis*) and PFMs act synergistically, it is necessary for them to relax together during urination and defecation.

The simplest way for children to learn how to relax their abdominal muscles is through diaphragmatic breathing exercises. During diaphragmatic breathing, in inspiration, the diaphragm moves caudally and pushes the abdominal organs forward. The anterior abdominal wall relaxes, as do the PFMs. This forward bulging of the anterior abdominal wall has been shown to reduce urethral pressure in healthy women and thus facilitate urination and defecation [58] .

Our institution was the first to incorporate this novel approach to treating DV. In a prospective clinical study of 43 children, in addition to standard urotherapy that included education on the importance of regular urination and hydration, proper voiding position and pattern, diaphragmatic breathing exercises and PFM relaxation exercises were performed in hospital settings for two weeks and then continued at home [60].

Diaphragmatic breathing exercises were performed in a supine position with the lower extremities supported by a pillow and hands placed on the abdominal muscles. The patient is required to inhale air through the nose, expel the anterior abdominal wall, hold the breath for a few seconds, and then exhale the air through the mouth (**Figures 4** and **5**). The exercises were repeated in both lateral positions, in the prone position, and then in the sitting position in front of the mirror (**Figure 6**). Children are required to observe the anterior abdominal wall during inspiration and then apply this exercise before urinating and defecating.

In addition, exercises for relaxation of the PFMs were performed. The child was placed in a lateral position with the upper leg flexed at the hip and knee and the lower leg extended. To enhance the proprioception of the PFMs, the examiner placed two fingers on the child's perineum and demanded that the child contract the PFMs without activating adjacent muscles such as the gluteus and hip adductor muscles. In this way, the child learned to localize and control the PFMs. The child was then required to perform submaximal contractions for 3 seconds followed by prolonged relaxation for about 30 seconds, for a total of 20 contractions. Children are required to perform these exercises daily at home for 6 months.

Control examinations were performed monthly for 12 months. Clinical manifestations (daytime urinary incontinence, nocturnal enuresis, urinary tract infections,

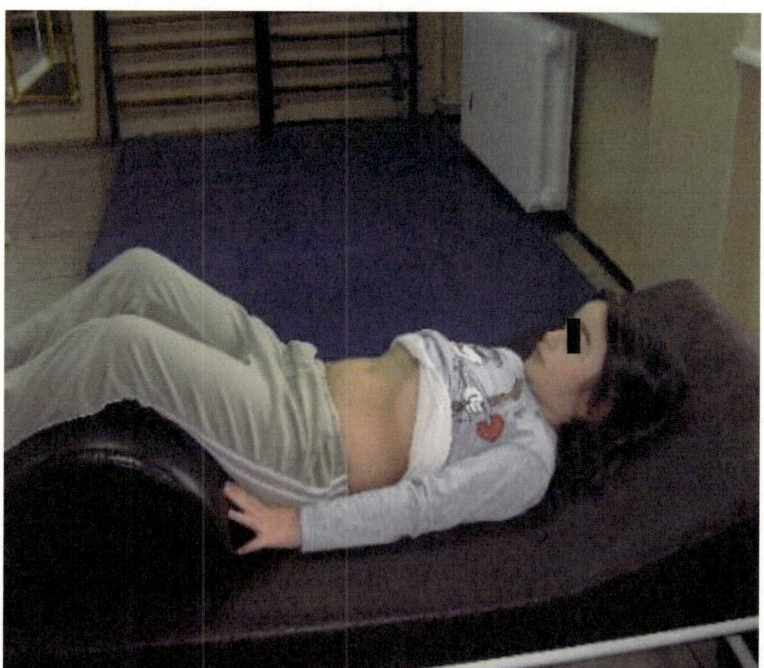

Figure 4.
Diaphragmatic breathing exercises in supine position (expiration).

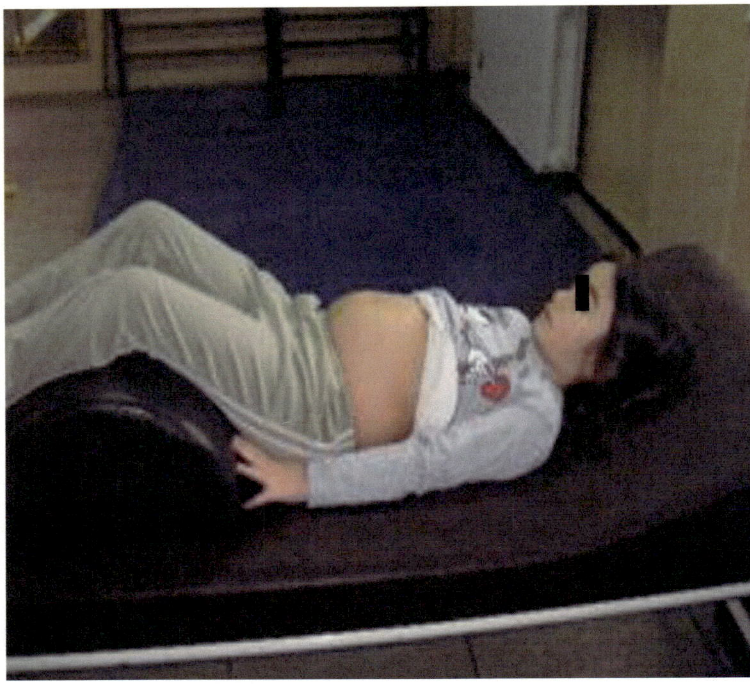

Figure 5.
Diaphragmatic breathing exercises in supine position (inspiration).

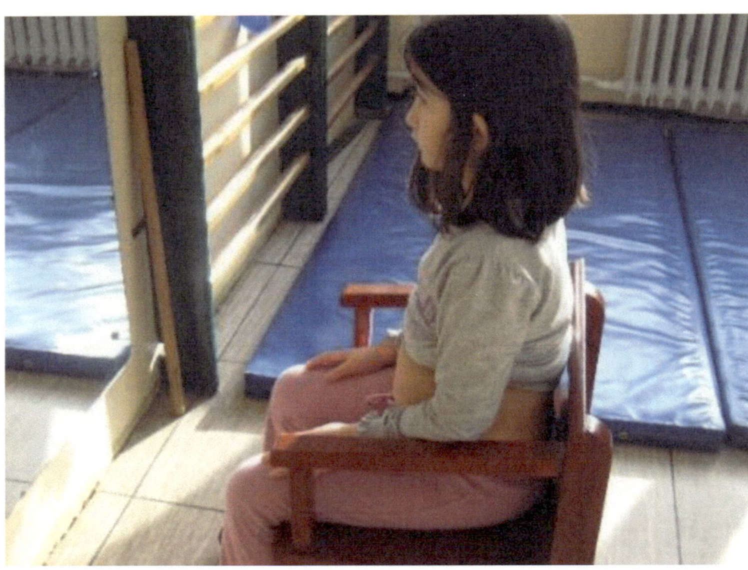

Figure 6.
Diaphagmatic breathing exercises in front of the mirror.

constipation) were analyzed on a monthly basis and uroflowmetry was performed. The performance of diaphragmatic breathing exercises was controlled and the importance of daily exercise at home was emphasized. The children are encouraged to continue with the treatment.

After one year of monitoring and treatment, reevaluation of clinical manifestations and uroflowmetry parameters was performed. Urinary incontinence was cured in 83% of children, nocturnal enuresis in 63%, and urinary tract infections in 68%. Chronic constipation was cured in all 15 patients. In addition, an objective improvement in uroflowmetry parameters was achieved. A normal uroflowmetry curve was registered in 90% of children.

The authors suggested that examination of lower abdominal muscles, recognition of their function during voiding and their relaxation should be incorporated in the treatment program of these children. Easy to learn diaphragmatic breathing exercises did not require any specific equipment and could be performed in children from five years of age. For centres that do not have access to pelvic floor EMG biofeedback, this programme could provide a treatment alternative as success rates are comparable to previous studies that used pelvic floor EMG biofeedback during urotherapy [54–56]. In order to achieve subjective and objective progress, children needed an average of 6.5 sessions, which is also equivalent to the average number of sessions in programmes that included non-animated biofeedback [46].

In the following study, the effects obtained in this group were compared with the effects in the group of children treated only with standard urotherapy (32 children) [31]. The children had 10 sessions of urotherapy in a hospital setting, and then were required to continue with it at home. After one year of follow-up, cure of urinary incontinence was achieved in only two children, nocturnal enuresis in 5, and urinary tract infections in 6 children. Constipation was cured in 6 out of 10 children. Uroflowmetry parameters did not show significant improvements. The authors concluded that diaphragmatic breathing exercises and PFM relaxation exercises, in combination with standard urotherapy, are important for the treatment of daily urinary incontinence, nocturnal enuresis and urinary tract infections, as well as for normalizing bladder function in children with DV.

5.4 Pharmacological therapy

Pharmacological therapy is considered an adjunct to improve bladder emptying in children with DV [43].

5.4.1 A-1 *adrenergic receptor blockers*

The role of α-1 adrenergic receptor blockers in the treatment of children with DV is controversial, as the mechanism of action at the level of the external urethral sphincter is still insufficiently known [61]. The possible mechanism of action is traditionally assumed to be relaxation of the periurethral, prostatic and bladder neck smooth muscles. In the study of Yucel et al., it has been shown that the effects of α-1 adrenergic blockers in reducing post-void residual urine can be compared with the effect of biofeedback [62].

5.4.2 Muscle relaxants

As DV is characterized by the inability of relaxation of the external urinary sphincter during urination, it was considered that muscle relaxant could be used in treatment.

Baclofen has been shown to be effective in reducing skeletal muscle spasticity, as well as in patients with striated sphincter dyssynergia [63]. However, the therapeutic effect is achieved only after the application of high doses. Serious adverse effects, especially after abrupt withdrawal, reduce its efficacy and safety in children with DV [64]. Therefore, tizanidine, a muscle relaxant used in many studies as a short-acting muscle relaxant due to spasmolytic action, was used. In a prospective, randomized study, 40 children with DV were divided into two groups [65]. The first group was treated with tizanidine (an imidazole derivative), while the second group of children was treated with α-blocker (doxazosin). After 6 months of follow-up, both groups had similar improvement in symptoms and uroflowmetry parameters. In the doxazosin-treated group, urgency was the only symptom that showed a significant reduction after therapy. However, nocturnal enuresis, urgency, and daytime incontinence were significantly reduced in the tizanidine-treated group. Side effects were reported in 6 patients (15%). Epigastric pain was reported in two children (10%) receiving doxazosin. In the tizanidin group, loss of appetite was noted in two children (10%), epigastric pain in one (5%) and headache in one child (5%).

5.5 Botulinum toxin type A (BT-A)

BT-A is one of the strongest known toxins. When injected directly into a muscle, it causes flaccid paralysis by blocking the presynaptic release of acetylcholine [66].

The use of BT-A in patients with detrusor sphincter dyssynergia (DSD) was first described by Dykstra et al. [67]. In this study, BT-A was injected into the external urinary sphincter of adult patients with spinal cord injury and DSD. Positive results, reduced urethral pressure, and volume of residual urine remained for an average of 50 days.

Indications for the injection of BT-A in the external urinary sphincter have been extended over time to adult patients with DV and detrusor hypocontractility. In the study by Kuo et al. clinical and urodynamic improvement was registered in 83% of patients with urethral sphincter non-relaxation and detrusor hypocontractility [68]. Petit and co-workers reported a significant reduction in detrusor and urethral pressure, as well as the volume of post-void residual urine after a single injection of 150 units Dysport (BT-A) in patients with spinal cord injury and DSD [69]. The beneficial effects of the therapy lasted for about 2-3 months.

In children treated with BT-A (amp. Dysport) due to spasticity, the most commonly reported adverse effects were local muscle weakness, urinary incontinence, fatigue, somnolence, flu-like symptoms, fever, and rash [70].

BT-A is used in the treatment of DV in children who are resistant to standard urotherapy. In the study of Radojicic et al., BT-A was applied in to the external urinary sphincter in children with DV [71]. The residual urine decreased significantly in 17 of 20 patients after 6 months of follow-up. The authors emphasized that temporary inhibition of the external urinary sphincter and/or PFMs may interrupt the DV cycle. The use of urotherapy during this period could help the child to re-adopt a normal urination pattern and thus reduce the need for re-injections.

In our institution, a prospective clinical study included 9 neurologically healthy girls with DV, aged 3-11 years, who had previously been treated with standard urotherapy without improvement [72]. Application of BT-A (amp. Dysport) in a dose of 500 units was performed transperineally into the external urethral sphincter. After two weeks of application, rehabilitation treatment consisting of standard urotherapy and PFM relaxation exercises was included. Six months after Dysport administration, there was a statistically significant improvement in clinical manifestations (urinary incontinence, voiding difficulties, urinary tract infections), and a significant reduction in post-void residual urine. No significant improvement in uroflowmetry parameters was registered. No children had systemic side effects with Dysport. The authors concluded that the act of urination in children with DV resistant to standard therapy can be significantly improved and maintained for at least 6 months after the use of amp. Dysport and urotherapy.

5.6 Manual physical therapy

Manual physical therapy with an osteopathic approach (MPT-OA) entails palpation and receptive manipulation of body tissues to relieve restraints that limit mobility and health. Biomechanical, myofascial, and articular constraints can contribute to DV by altering alignment, distorting the pelvis, restricting mobility, and thus affecting pressures within the abdominal and pelvic cavities [73]. Altered pressure relationships can affect neurological, vascular, lymphatic, and hormonal functions. In the randomized controlled trial that involved 21 children with DV, it has been shown that children with additional 4 sessions of MPT-OA demonstrated better short-term results compared to children that had only standard treatment [73]. The authors speculated that MPT-OA treatment helped restoring more natural alignment and mobility which helped the abdominal and PFMs to function more efficiently. However this single-centre promising results should be confirmed by multi-centre randomized controlled trials in order to draw definitive conclusions of MPT-OA in children with DV.

6. Conclusion

Urotherapy is the cornerstone of DV care for children. The treatment begins with standard urotherapy, after which specific measures are added. Rehabilitation programmes with diaphragmatic breathing exercises and pelvic floor relaxation exercises are superior in curing lower urinary tract symptoms and normalizing urinary function than programmes that only include standard urotherapy. The success rates of programmes that included pelvic floor relaxation exercises and diaphragmatic breathing exercises without the use of pelvic floor EMG biofeedback were equivalent to those that included pelvic floor EMG biofeedback, proposing a treatment choice for centres that do not have access to EMG biofeedback. However, no standardized pelvic floor exercise protocol egists. Therefore, new prospective multicentric randomized trials with a larger number of children are needed to determine the most appropriate programme that will have the best therapeutic outcome.

Acknowledgements

This work has been supported by the Ministry of Science and Technological Development of the Republic of Serbia, under the project 43011.

Conflict of interest

None declared.

Author details

Vesna D. Zivkovic[1,2*], Ivona Stankovic[1,2], Lidija Dimitrijevic[1,2], Hristina Colovic[1,2], Dragan Zlatanovic[1,2] and Natasa Savic[3]

1 Faculty of Medicine, University of Nis, Nis, Serbia

2 Clinic of Physical Medicine and Rehabilitation, University Clinical Centre, Nis, Serbia

3 College of Health Studies Cuprija, Cuprija, Serbia

*Address all correspondence to: petvesna67@gmail.com

References

[1] Gontard A, Neveus T. Introduction. In: Hart M (ed). Management of disorders of bladder and bowel control in childhood. London: Mac Keith Press; 2006. p. 1-2.

[2] Sillen U. Epidemiology. In: Proceedings of the ICCS course on„ Multidisciplinary management of nocturnal and diurnal wetting problems in children" & ESPU course on„Surgery for the incontinent child and bowel problems"; 14-17 September Antalya, Turkey, 2006. p. 136-40.

[3] Hjalmas K, Arnold T, Bower W, Caione P,Chiozza LM, von Gontard A, et al. Nocturnal enuresis: an international evidence based management strategy. J Urol 2004;171:2545-61. doi: 10.1097/01.ju.0000111504.85822.b2

[4] Austin PF, Bauer SB, Bower W, Chase J, Franco I, Hoebeke P et al. The standardization of terminology of lower urinary tract function in children and adolescents: Update Report from the standardization committee of the International Children's Continence Society. Neurourol Urodyn. 2016; 35(4):471-81. doi: 10.1002/nau.22751

[5] Hinman F, Baumann FW. Vesical and ureteral damage from voiding dysfunction in boys without neurologic or obstructive disease. J Urol 1973;109:727-32. doi: 10.1016/s0022-5347(17)60526-3.

[6] Von Gontard A. Enuresis im Kindesalter – psychiatrische, somatische und molekulargenetische Zusammenhange [thesis]. Keln: Universitat zu Koln; 1995.

[7] Hoang-Bohm J, Lusch A, Sha W, Alken P. Biofeedback for urinary bladder dysfunctions in childhood. Indications, practice and the results of therapy. Urologe A 2004;43:813-9. doi: 10.1007/s00120-004-0617-3.

[8] Hoebeke P, Van Laecke AR, Van Camp C, Raes A, Van De Walle J. One thousand video-urodynamic studies in children with non-neurogenic bladder sphincter dysfunction. BJU Int 2001; 87(6): 575-80. doi: 10.1046/j.1464-410x.2001.00083.

[9] Burgers RE, Mugie SM, Chase J, Cooper CS, von Gontard A, Rittig CS et al. Management of functional constipation in children with lower urinary tract symptoms: Report from the standardization committee of the International Children's Continence Society. J Urol. 2013; 190: 29-36. doi: 10.1016/j.juro.2013.01.001

[10] Allen TD. The nonneurogenic neurogenic bladder. J Urol 1977;117:23. doi: 10.1016/s0022-5347(17)58412-8

[11] Van Gool JD, Kuitjen RH, Donckerwolcke RA, Messer AP, Vijverberg M. Bladder-sphincter dysfunction, urinary infection and vesico-uretheral reflux with special reference to cognitive bladder training. Contrib Nephrol 1984;39: 190-210. doi: 10.1159/000409249.

[12] Hjalmas K. Is dyscoordinated voiding in children an hereditary disorder. Scand J Urol Nephrol Suppl 1995;173:31-5.

[13] Koff S, Jayanthi V. Non-neurogenic lower urinary tract dysfunction. In: Walsh PC, Retik AB, Vaughn ED, Wein AJ (eds). Cambell's Urology. 8th Ed. Philadelphia: WB Saunders Co; 2002. p. 2262-83.

[14] Vijverberg MAW, Elzinga-Plomp A, Messer AP, van Gool JD, de Jong TP. Bladder rehabilitation, the effect of cognitive training programme on urge incontinence. Eur Urol 1997 ;31:68-72. doi: 10.1159/000474421.

[15] Wiener JS, Scales MT, Hampton J, King LR, Surwit R, Edwards CL.

Long-term efficacy of simple behavioral therapy for daytime wetting in children. J Urol 2000; 164 (3 pt 1): 786-90. doi: 10.1097/00005392-200009010-00048.

[16] Bakker E, van Gool JD, van Sprudel M, King LR, Surwit R, Edwards CL. Results of a questionnaire evaluating the effects of different method of toilet training on achieving bladder control. BJU int 2002;90:456-61. doi: 10.1097/00005392-200009010-00048.

[17] Cooper C, Abousally C, Austin C, Boyt M, Hawtrey C. Do public schools teach voiding dysfunction? Results of an school teacher survey. J Urol 2003;170:956-8. doi: 10.1097/01.ju.0000075916.55446.ee.

[18] Ellsworth P, Merguerian P, Copening ME. Sexual Abuse: Another causative factor in dysfunctional voiding. J Urol 1995;153:773-6.

[19] Vincent SA. Postural control of urinary incontinence. The curtsey sign. Lancet 1966; 2 (7464) : 631-2. doi: 10.1016/s0140-6736(66)91942-8.

[20] Koff SA, Wagner TT, Jayanthi VR. The relationship among dysfunctional elimination syndromes, primary vesicoureteral reflux and urinary tract infections in children. J Urol 1998;160:1019-22. doi: 10.1097/00005392-199809020-00014.

[21] McKenna LS, McKenna PH. Modern management of nonneurologic pediatric incontinence. J WOCN 2004; 31(6): 351-6. doi: 10.1097/00152192-200411000-00006.

[22] Hoebeke P. Voiding dysfunction, recurrent UTI, constipation, and vesicoureteric reflux: a common disease complex. In: Fourth course on paediatric urodynamics, Utrecht. Edited by European Society of Paediatric Urology, 2005. p. 61-5.

[23] Kaufman JJ. A new recording uroflowmeter: a simple automatic device for measuring voiding velocity. J Urol 1957;78:97-9. doi: 10.1016/s0022-5347(17)66405

[24] Hellstrom AL, Hjalmas K, Jodal U. Rehabilitation of the dysfunctional bladder in children: method and 3-year follow-up. J Urol 1987; 138:847-9. doi: 10.1016/s0022-5347(17)43395-7.

[25] De Paepe H, Renson C, Hoebeke P, Raes A, Van Laecke E, Vande Walle J. The role of pelvic-floor therapy in the treatment of lower urinary tract dysfunctions in children. Scand J Urol Nephrol 2002; 36(4): 260-7. doi: 10.1080/003655902320248218.

[26] Wennergren HM, Oberg BE, Sandstedt P. Importance of leg support for relaxation of the pelvic floor muscles. A surface electromyographic study in healthy girls. Scand J Urol Nephrol 1991;25:205-13. doi: 10.3109/00365599109107948

[27] Mugie SM, Di Lorenco C, Benninga MA. Constipation in childhood. Nat Rev Gastroenterol Hepatol 2011;8:502-11. doi: 10.1038/nrgastro.2011.130.

[28] Bongers ME, van Wijk MP, Reitsma JB, Benninga MA. Long-term prognosis for childhood constipation: clinical outcomes in adulthood. Pediatrics. 2010;126(1):e156-62. doi: 10.1542/peds.2009-1009.

[29] Van Dijk M, Bongers ME, de Vries GJ, Grootenhuis MA, Last BF, Benninga MA. Behavioral therapy for childhood constipation: a randomized, controlled trial. Pediatrics. 2008; 121(5):e1334-41. doi: 10.1542/peds.2007-2402.

[30] Van Dijk M, Benninga MA, Grootenhuis MA, Nieuwenhuizen AM, Last BF. Chronic childhood constipation: a review of the literature

and the introduction of a protocolized behavioral intervention program. Patient Educ Couns. 2007; 67: 63-77. doi: 10.1016/j.pec.2007.02.002.

[31] Zivkovic V, Lazovic M, Stankovic I, Vlajkovic M, Slavkovic A. The evaluation of combined standard urotherapy, abdominal and pelvic floor retraining in children with dysfunctional voiding. J Pediatr Urol. 2011; 7: 336-41. doi: 10.1016/j.jpurol.2011.02.028.

[32] Kajbafzadeh AM, LidaSharifi-Rad L, Ghahestani SM, Ahmadi H, Kajbafzadeh M, Mahboubiet AH. Animated biofeedback: an ideal treatment for children with dysfunctional elimination syndrome. J Urol. 2011; 186: 2379-84. doi: 10.1016/j.juro.2011.07.118.

[33] Loening-Baucke V. Modulation of abnormal defaecation dynamics by biofeedback treatment in chronically constipated children with encopresis. J Pediatr. 1990; 116:214-22. doi: 10.1016/s0022-3476(05)82877-x.

[34] Zivkovic VD, Stankovic I, Dimitrijevic L, Kocic M, Colovic H, Vlajkovic M, et al. Are interferential electrical stimulation and diaphragmatic breathing exercises beneficial in children with bladder and bowel dysfunction? Urology 2017; 102: 207-12. doi: 10.1016/j.urology.2016.12.038.

[35] Savic N, Zivkovic V, Stankovic I, Stojkovic T, Milenkovic M, Stojanovic Z, Balov B. The role of physical therapy in the treatment of children with chronic functional constipation. Military-Medical and Pharmaceutical Review 2020;77:87-91. doi: 10.2298/VSP170503039S.

[36] Keshtgar AS, Ward HC, Clayden GS. Transcutaneous needle-free injection of botulinum toxin: a novel treatment of childhood constipation and anal fissure. J Pediatr Surg. 2009; 44: 1791-98. doi: 10.1016/j.jpedsurg.2009.02.056.

[37] Leong LC, Yik YI, Catto-Smith AG, Robertson VJ, Hutson JM, Southwell BR. Long-term effects of transabdominal electrical stimulation in treating children with slow-transit constipation. J Pediatr Surg. 2011; 46: 2309-12. doi: 10.1016/j.jpedsurg.2011.09.022.

[38] Clarke MC, Chase JW, Gibb S, Robertson VJ, Catto-Smith A, Hutson JM, Southwell BR. Decreased colonic transit time after transcutaneous interferential electrical stimulation in children with slow transit constipation. J Pediatr Surg. 2009; 44: 408-12. doi: 10.1016/j.jpedsurg.2008.10.100.

[39] Chase J, Robertson VJ, Southwell B, Hutson J, Gibb S. Pilot study using transcutaneous electrical stimulation (interferential current) to treat chronic treatment-resistant constipation and soiling in children. J Gastroenterol Hepatol. 2005; 20: 1054-61. doi: 10.1111/j.1440-1746.2005.03863.x.

[40] Wennerrgren H, Oberg B. Pelvic floor exercises for children: A method of treating dysfunctional voiding. BJU 1995;76:9-15. doi: 10.1111/j.1464-410x.1995.tb07823.x.

[41] Maizels M, King LR, Firlit CF. Urodynamic biofeedback: a new approach to treat vesical sphincter dyssynergia. J Urol. 1979;122:205-209.

[42] Kjolseth D, Knudsen LM, Madsen B, Nørgaard JP, Djurhuus JC. Urodynamic biofeedback training for children with bladder-sphincter-discoordination during voiding. Neurourol Urodyn 1993;12:211-21. doi: 10.1002/nau.1930120303.

[43] Chase J, Austin P, Hoebeke P, McKenna P. The management of dysfunctional voiding in children: A report from the standardisation committee of the International

Children's Continence Society. J Urol 2010;183: 1296-302. doi: 10.1016/j.juro.2009.12.059.

[44] McKenna PH, Herndon CD, Connery S, Ferrer FA. Pelvic-floor muscle retraining for paediatric voiding dysfunction using interactive computer games. J Urol 1999; 162 (3 pt 2): 1056-63.

[45] Herndon A, Decambre M, McKenna P. Interactive computer games for treatment of pelvic floor dysfunction. J Urol 2001;166:1893-98.

[46] Kaye JD, Palmer LS. Animated biofeedback yields more rapid results than nonanimated biofeedback in the treatment of dysfunctional voiding in girls. J Urol. 2008;180:300-5. doi: 10.1016/j.juro.2008.03.078.

[47] Desantis DJ, Leonard MP, Preston MA, Barrowman NJ, Guerra LA. Effectiveness of biofeedback for dysfunctional elimination syndrome in pediatrics: a systematic review. J Pediatr Urol. 2011;7:342-48. doi: 10.1016/j.jpurol.2011.02.019.

[48] Palmer LS, Franco I, Rotario P, Reda EF, Friedman SC, Kolligian ME, et al. Biofeedback therapy expedites the resolution of reflux in older children. J Urol. 2002;168(4 Pt 2):1699-1702. doi: 10.1097/01.ju.0000028012.24758.33.

[49] Khen-Dunlop N, Van Egroo A, Bouteiller C, Bouteiller C, Biserte J, Besson R. Biofeedback therapy in the treatment of bladder overactivity, vesico-ureteral reflux and urinary tract infection. J Pediatr Urol. 2006;2:424-29.

[50] Kibar Y, Ors O, Demir E, Kalman S, Sakallioglu O, Dayanc M. Results of biofeedback treatment on reflux resolution rates in children with dysfunctional voiding and vesicoureteral reflux. Urology. 2007;70:563-66. doi: 10.1016/j.jpurol.2005.09.004.

[51] Palmer LS. Evaluation and targeted therapy of voiding dysfunction in children. Urology. 2016;92:87-94. doi: 10.1016/j.urology.2016.02.002

[52] De Paepe H, Renson C, van Laecke AR, Raes A, Vande Walle J, Hoebeke P. Pelvic-floor therapy and toilet training in young children with dysfunctional voiding and obstipation. BJU Int 2000; 85(7): 889-93. doi: 10.1046/j.1464-410x.2000.00664.x.

[53] Vasconcelos M, Lima E, Caiafa L, Noronha A, Cangussu R, Gomes S et al. Voiding dysfunction in children. Pelvic floor exercises or biofeedback therapy: a randomized study. Pediatric Nephrol 2006; 21: 1858-64. doi: 10.1007/s00467-006-0277-1.

[54] Shei DeiYang S, Wang CC. Outpatient biofeedback relaxation of the pelvic floor in treating pediatric dysfunctional voiding: a short-course program is effective. Urol Int 2005; 74:118-22. doi: 10.1159/000083281.

[55] Yagci S, Kibar Y, Akay O, Kilic S, Erdemir F, Gok F, Dayanc M. The effect of biofeedback treatment on voiding and urodynamic parameters in children with voiding dysfunction. J Urol 2005; 174: 1994-7. doi: 10.1097/01.ju.0000176487.64283.36.

[56] Drzewiecki BA, Kelly PR, Marinaccio B, Borer JG, Estrada CR, Lee RS, Bauer SB. Biofeedback training for lower urinary tract symptoms: factors affecting efficacy. J Urol 2009; 182: 2050-5. doi: 10.1016/j.juro.2009.06.003.

[57] Sapsford R. Rehabilitation of pelvic floor muscles utilizing trunk stabilization. Manual Therapy 2004; 9:3-12. doi: 10.1016/s1356-689x(03)00131-0.

[58] Sapsford RR, Hodges PW. Contraction of pelvic floor muscles during abdominal maneuvers. Arch

Phys Med Rehab 2001;82:1081-8. doi: 10.1053/apmr.2001.24297.

[59] Sapsford RR, Hodges PV, Richardson CA, Cooper DH, Markwell SJ, Jull GA. Co-activation of abdominal and pelvic floor muscles during voluntary exercises. Neurourol Urodyn 2001; 20: 31-42. doi: 10.1002/1520-6777(2001)20:1<31::aid-nau5>3.0.co;2-p.

[60] Zivkovic V, Lazovic M, Vlajkovic M, Slavkovic A, Dimitrijevic L, Stankovic I, Vacic N. The role of diaphragmatic breathing exercises and pelvic floor retraining in children with dysfunctional voiding. Eur J Phys Rehab Med 2012;48:413-21.

[61] Kramer SA, Rathbun SR, Elkins D, Karnes RJ, Husmann DA. Double-blind placebo controlled study of α-adrenergic receptor antagonists (doxazosin) for treatment of voiding dysfunction in pediatric pupulation. J Urol 2005; 173(6):2121-4. doi: 10.1097/01.ju.0000157689.98314.69.

[62] Yucel S, Akkaya E, Guntekin E, Kukul E, Akman S, Melikoglu M, Baykara M. Can alpha-blocker therapy be an alternative to biofeedback for dysfunctional voiding and urinary retention? A prospective study. J Urol 2005;174(4 pt 2): 1612-5. doi: 10.1097/01.ju.0000179241.99381.5e.

[63] Cedarbaum JM, Schleifer LS. Drugs for Parkinson's disease, spasticity and acute muscle spasms. In: Rall TW, Nies AS, Taylor P, eds. Goodman and Gilman's the Pharmacological Basis of Therapeutics, 8th ed. New York: Pergamon; 1990. p. 463-84.

[64] Palazón García R, Benavente Valdepeñas A, Arroyo Riaño O. Protocol for tizanidine use in infantile cerebral palsy. Ann Paediatr. 2008;68:511-515. doi: 10.1157/13120053.

[65] El-Hefnawy AS, Helmy T, El-Assmy MM, Sarhan O, Hafez AT, Dawaba M. Doxazosin versus tizanidine for treatment of dysfunctional voiding in children: a prospective randomized open-labeled trial. Urology 2012;79: 428-433. doi: 10.1016/j.urology.2011.10.043.

[66] Riccabona M, Koen M, Schindler M, Goedele B, Pycha A, Lusuardi L, Bauer SB. Botulinum-A toxin injection into the detrusor: a safe alternative in the treatment of children with myelomeningocele with detrusor hyperreflexia. J Urol 2004: 171;845-48. doi: 10.1097/01.ju.0000108892.35041.2d.

[67] Dykstra DD, Sidi AA, Scott AB, Pagel JM, Goldish GD. Effects of Botulinum-A toxin on detrusor-sphincter dyssynergia in spinal cord injury patients. J Urol 1988: 139;919-22. doi: 10.1016/s0022-5347(17)42717-0.

[68] Kuo HC. Effect of botulinum A toxin in the treatment of voiding dysfunction due to detrusor underactivity. Urology 2003: 61;550-54. doi: 10.1016/s0090-4295(02)02541-4.

[69] Petit H, Wiart L, Gaujard E, Le Breton F, Ferrière JM, Lagueny A, et al. Botulinum-A toxin treatment for detrusor-sphincter dyssynergia in spinal cord disease. Spinal Cord 1998: 36;91-94. doi: 10.1038/sj.sc.3100517.

[70] Bakheit AMO, Severa S, Cosgrove A, Morton R, Roussounis SH, Doderlein L, Lin JP. Safety profile and efficacy of Botulinum toxin A (Dysport) in children with muscle spasticity. Dev Med Child Neurol 2001: 43; 234-38. doi: 10.1017/s0012162201000445.

[71] Radojicic Z, Perovic S, Milic N. Is it reasonable to treat refractory voiding dysfunction in children with Botulinum-A toxin. J Urol 2006:176; 332-36. doi: 10.1016/S0022-5347(06)00298-9.

[72] Petronijevic V, Lazovic M, Vlajkovic M, Slavkovic A, Golubovic E,

Miljkovic P. Botulinum toxin type A in combination with standard urotherapy for children with dysfunctional voiding. J Urol 2007; 178(6): 2599-603. doi: 10.1016/j.juro.2007.08.027.

[73] Nemett DR, Fivush BA, Mathews R, Camirand N, Eldridge MA, Finney K, Gerson AC. A randomized controlled trial of the effectiveness of osteopathy-based manual physical therapy in treating pediatric dysfunctional voiding. J Pediatr Urol. 2008 Apr;4(2):100-6. doi: 10.1016/j.jpurol.2007.11.006.

Chapter 8

Surgical Treatment of Pelvic Organ Prolapse

Cristina Margarita Fernández-Ávila,
Rodrigo García-Baquero, Ana Victoria Ojeda Claro,
Blanca Madurga Patuel and José Luis Álvarez-Ossorio

Abstract

The human being is the only mammal capable of walking and simultaneously maintaining an upright position. This fact, implies somewhat unfavorable repercussions for the pelvic region that must support the weight of the abdominal organs. A prime example of the aforementioned adverse effects of the standing position are pelvic organ prolapses (POP). POP surgery is an increasingly important therapeutic aspect in clinical practice due to the aging of our population, and is increasingly prevalent as a therapeutic option. Surgical techniques can be performed using an abdominal or vaginal approach, depending on the medical history, physical examination, and experience of the surgeon. Laparoscopic sacrocolpopexy is an adequate therapeutic option with a high success rate in 80–100% of cases. However, this technique is not always appropriate, especially for patients who are at high risk for anesthesia, a multi-operated abdomen, or in recurrent prolapse. In these cases, a vaginal approach offers an interesting surgical alternative. In this review, we added our experience with transvaginal single-incision mesh under locoregional anesthesia for correction of female POP. We retrospectively analyzed 78 patients showing a success rate of 92% after more than 12 months of follow up. Transvaginal mesh was developed to maintain the advantage of a vaginal procedure, while reducing the risk of recurrent prolapse compared to native tissue repair and simplifying the surgery compared to sacrocolpopexy.

Keywords: Pelvic Organ Prolapse, Reconstructive Surgical Procedures, Gynecologic Surgical Procedures

1. Introduction

The human being is the only mammal capable of walking and simultaneously maintaining an upright position. This fact, greatly affected by the law of gravity, implies somewhat unfavorable repercussions for the pelvic region that must support the weight of the abdominal organs. Therefore, throughout evolution, fundamental modifications have emerged in the pelvic skeleton, and in the surrounding muscles and ligaments, to offset the negative effect of the law of gravity. A prime example of the aforementioned adverse effects of the standing position are pelvic organ prolapses (POP).

The prevalence of this pathology is clearly on the rise: it is estimated that the number of women with pelvic organ prolapse will rise from 3.3 million women in 2010 to 4.9 million in 2050. Pelvic floor dysfunction is considered to be underdiagnosed, affecting 50% of women, although only 10–20% will seek assistance [1]. More than 60% of the patients affected by this condition present more than one pathology as the pelvic floor organs constitute a functional and organic unit [2]. It is estimated that a woman's risk of undergoing surgery related with POP during her life varies from 6.3 to 19%, with 30% requiring one or more surgical interventions due to recurrence [3]. Some authors have reported re-intervention rates for recurrence after primary reconstructive surgery of between 43 and 58% [4].

The anatomical support of the pelvic viscera is provided mainly by the levator ani and the connective tissue junctions of the pelvic organs: vaginal support arises from the connective tissue junctions between the vagina and the pelvic lateral wall, the vaginal wall and levator ani muscles [5].

In 1994, Delancey had already introduced the concept of the division of the support of the pelvic connective tissue in three levels (I-III) that represent apical, mid-vaginal and distal support, respectively. The upper portion of the paracolpium (Level I) consists of a lamina from which the vagina is suspended attaching it to the pelvic wall, and is responsible for suspending the apex of the vagina after hysterectomy. In the middle third of the vagina, the paracolpium joins the vagina laterally to the tendinous arch and the fascia of the elevator ani muscles (Level II). This stretches the vagina transversally between the bladder and the rectum. The structural layer that supports the bladder (pubocervical fascia) is made up of the anterior vaginal region and its attachment through the endopelvic fascia to the pelvic wall. Similarly, the posterior vaginal wall and endopelvic fascia (rectovaginal fascia) form the containing layer that prevents protrusion of the rectum toward its anterior surface. The lower third of the vagina (Level III) fuses with the perineal membrane, levator ani muscle, and the perineal body. Defects in the mid-level vaginal base (pubocervical and rectovaginal fascia) result in cystocele and rectocele, while the loss of upper suspensory fibers of the paracolpium and parametrium are responsible for the development of vaginal and uterine prolapse, and these defects of combined form [6].

During examination, the prolapse of the anterior compartment is the most frequently reported site of prolapse and it is diagnosed twice as frequently as the defects of the posterior compartment, and three times more common than apical prolapse [7]. After hysterectomy, 6–12% of women will develop a prolapse of the vaginal vault [8] and in two thirds, multi-compartmental prolapse will be present.

The etiology of POP is believed to be multi-factorial with contributions from both environmental and genetic risk factors. The environmental factors that contribute to POP include vaginal delivery and newborn weight, chronic increases in intra-abdominal pressure, obesity, advanced age and estrogen deficiency [9].

Not all prolapses are clinically symptomatic, and finding mild asymptomatic prolapses during pelvic floor examination is common. If symptoms are present, the most frequent complaints include a sensation of pressure, a lump or protrusion and with evidence upon physical examination of a second degree or greater anterior and / or posterior and / or central vaginal wall prolapse. Ellerkmann et al. found that in 237 women evaluated for POP, 73% reported urinary incontinence, 86% urinary urgency and / or frequency, 34–62% voiding dysfunction and 31% fecal incontinence [10]. Evaluation of a patient with vaginal prolapse requires a comprehensive review of the full spectrum of pelvic floor symptoms and an assessment of how these symptoms affect her quality of life.

2. Surgical treatment of pelvic organ prolapse

POP surgery is an increasingly important therapeutic aspect in clinical practice due to the aging of our population, and is increasingly prevalent as a therapeutic option, despite surgical and hospitalization times that are three times longer compared to other surgeries related to the pelvic floor such as continence surgery. Given the increasing time and resources that will be required for POP surgery in the future, it is paramount that we perform effective, long-lasting and cost-effective interventions with minimal morbidity.

Historically, most studies evaluating the treatment of POP have focused exclusively on anatomic success without considering other important aspects such as symptoms, vaginal accommodation, and quality of life. In fact, for a patient, individually, the most important result of a surgical procedure is the relief of their symptoms and improvement of their quality of life [11]. However, until recently these areas have been ignored. The objectives of pelvic floor reconstruction are to relieve symptoms, restore anatomy, improve or preserve function, prevent actions that alter other compartments, and improve quality of life [12].

Anterior colporrhaphy was the standard procedure in the management of the prolapsed anterior compartment. That said in the early 2000s, there was a movement toward the use of prosthetics to increase the efficacy of native tissue repair in reconstructive gynecology. This was due to the articles published by Olsen et al. [13] where they reported a reoperation rate of 29% after prolapse or continence surgery and Weber et al. [14] who reported a 70% failure rate of native tissue anterior compartment repair. Recent reassessment of the same demographic 10 years later revealed a significantly lower reoperation rate of 17% [15]. More importantly, Weber et al. [14] and Sand et al. [16] reported in randomized controlled clinical trials that anterior colporrhaphy was successful in managing cystocele in only 30%. A recent re-analysis of the latter data, using the hymen as the threshold for objective success, reported considerably better results, with only 10% anatomic recurrence beyond the hymen, 5% symptomatic recurrence, and a lower reoperation rate of 1% at 23 months of follow-up [17]. During the decade between these initial and later publications, surgeons introduced a large number of biologic and mesh grafts to improve the outcomes of prolapse surgery. In later studies such as that of Julian et al. [18] it was shown that patients with several vaginal repairs had better results with a new repair with prosthetic material, in this case a Marlex® mesh (Bard, Covington, GA), compared to previous colporrhaphy, although follow-up reported an erosion rate of up to 25%.

The 2016 Cochrane Review also reported on 16 trials that evaluated nearly 2,000 women with the aim of comparing anterior colporrhaphy versus permanent polypropylene mesh POP repair. The meta-analysis showed that recurrence of anterior wall prolapse (RR 0.34, 95% CI 0.25 to 0.46) and reoperation for prolapse (RR 0.44, 95% CI 0.24 to 0.46) were significantly less common after mesh repair compared to colporrhaphy. There were no differences between the groups in terms of quality of life outcomes or dyspareunia rates. However, the transvaginal polypropylene mesh group had higher rates of reoperation due to mesh exposure, stress urinary incontinence or prolapse (RR 1.62, 95% CI 1.15 to 2.28), and prolapse in the apical or posterior compartment (RR 1.85, 95% CI 1.01 to 3.37) compared to anterior colporrhaphy. Surgical time (MD 17.9 min, 95% CI 10.0 to 25.8), transfusion rate (RR 2.37, 95% CI 1.32 to 4.24), cystotomy (RR 4.65, 95% CI 1.22 to 17.77) and de novo stress urinary incontinence (RR 1.55, 95% CI 1.02 to 2.35) were higher after use of transvaginal polypropylene mesh compared to colporrhaphy. The mesh erosion rate was 11.5% and 7% underwent surgical correction for repair [19].

One fact that we must take into account is that recently, most of the products made with polypropylene meshes evaluated in this meta-analysis have been withdrawn by the manufacturers due to the ongoing litigation regarding the use of this type of material vaginally. Because of this, new transvaginal polypropylene prosthetic products have emerged that have been introduced to decrease the rate of complications, specifically mesh erosion. Altman et al. [20] based on a multicenter prospective case series, which evaluated 207 women with apical prolapse undergoing the Uphold® pelvic floor system (Boston Scientific, USA), reported a subjective success rate of 90% per year and a reoperation rate for mesh exposure of 1.3%. Similarly, De Tayrac et al. [21] found at 3 years, in 79 women with grade 3–4 cystocele, an anatomical success rate of 95%, a satisfaction rate of 98% and a mesh exposure rate of 1.3% using a mesh of lightweight (28 g / m2) polypropylene (Surgimesh® Prolapse Xlight, Aspide Medical, France) [21].

Studies where the device used was Restorelle® (Coloplast, Minneapolis, USA), report rates of absence of postoperative complications of 98.2%. The most frequent complications included urinary retention (8.7%), urinary tract infections (5.5%), and hematoma (2.7%). Other complications related to neighboring organs (bladder, rectum, and ureters) were very rare (<1%). A total of 2.8% of the patients had grade III complications according to the Clavien-Dindo classification (mesh extrusion). 80.3% did not present complications during the 3 months of study follow-up. Despite these promising data, the follow-up time of this study is short to ensure the absence of complications within a longer follow-up period [22]. Despite the current negative sentiment around transvaginal mesh, these new lightweight mesh products require further reassessment.

In the 2016 Cochrane meta-analysis of grafts vs. Native tissue repairs for vaginal prolapse, only one case of reoperation for dyspareunia or pain was reported in the nearly 1000 cases of transvaginal mesh evaluated [19]. However, pain and dyspareunia were the main causes of adverse events that triggered the 2011 FDA (Food and Drug Administration) warnings on the safety of transvaginal mesh [23]. These findings raise the possibility that pain and dyspareunia after transvaginal mesh surgery may be underreported, and possibly only identified in trials with longer term evaluation.

Alternatively, autologous material was considered as a possible option to synthetic prosthetic grafts with a lower risk of host rejection or infection. Gandhi et al. reported preliminary results of a randomized control trial comparing anterior colporrhaphy alone vs. fascia lata graft for cystoceles [24]. In 1 year they could not demonstrate that the addition of the fascia lata graft improved the success rate compared to anterior colporrhaphy alone, being 71% compared to 82% (p 0.07), however, the rate of recurrent anterior prolapse in examination was lower after biological graft repair compared to anterior colporrhaphy (RR 0.74, 95% CI 0.55 to 0.99 n = 646, I2 = 29%, low-quality evidence), being the operative time for colporrhaphy shorter than the biological graft procedure (MD -10.35, 95% CI -14.45 to −6.24).

Reoperation after POP surgery for recurrence is an important measure of the effectiveness of the procedure. It is important to note that reoperation rates represent the "tip of the iceberg" in terms of surgical failures, as there are women with recurrent symptomatic prolapse who do not wish to undergo another operation. However, repeat surgery for recurrent POP is always an undesirable result that should, in most cases, be considered as a failed surgical procedure. Reoperation rates after POP surgery vary widely in the literature, largely due to different definitions and timelines. In a meta-analysis of 258 studies evaluating the reoperation rate after apical prolapse repairs, Diwadkar et al. reported a reoperation rate of 3.9% (95% CI: 3.5–4.4%) for traditional vaginal vault suspensions (sacrospinal ligament suspension and uterosacral vault suspensions) after a mean of 32 months, 2.3% (95% CI 1.9–2.7%) for sacrocolpopexy with follow-up mean 26 months and 1.3% (95% CI 1.0–1.7%) after transvaginal mesh procedures with a mean follow-up of 17 months. In particular, the total reoperation rate, including reoperations for recurrent POP and complications, was higher in the transvaginal mesh group (8.5%) [25].

The reoperation rate after POP surgery was defined in the joint report by the ICS (International Continence Society) and the IUGA (International Urogynecological Association), making a clear distinction between additional surgeries after primary surgical correction of POP, as the character of these can be very heterogeneous. The classification of these surgeries was established as follows:

- Primary prolapse / different compartment surgery - prolapse in a new compartment after previous surgery in a different compartment.

- Repeat surgery - is a repeat operation for prolapse that arises from the compartment that was previously operated on.

- Surgery for complications (e.g. exposure or extrusion of the mesh, pain, or hemodynamic compromise of the patient, hemorrhage).

- Surgery for conditions not related to prolapse (e.g. subsequent surgery for stress urinary incontinence or fecal incontinence).

Recently, Ow et al. retrospectively compared 237 women who underwent 185 native tissue repairs and 161 transvaginal mesh repairs for recurrent prolapse. The transvaginal mesh group had significantly lower follow-up rates of symptomatic prolapse, prolapse upon examination, and reoperation for prolapse, than the native tissue repairs group. However, the mesh exposure rate (anterior 15%, posterior mesh 21%) and associated reoperation (anterior 9%, posterior 15%) were significantly higher [26]. Trials such as this one show that in women with recurrent prolapse, transvaginal mesh has significant advantages and disadvantages compared to native tissue repairs and this profile is similar to that described for primary repairs, except that the exposure rates of the mesh appear to be higher in recurrent POP surgery.

Another surgical alternative on the rise in the last decade is laparoscopic or robotic sacrocolpopexy. This was born with the purpose of maintaining the existing good results of abdominal sacrocolpopexy but with the advantages of minimally invasive surgery. The case series demonstrate adequate acceptance in the short and medium term, with success rates of 91% (range 60–100%), subjective success rates of 79–98% [27, 28] and a mean reoperation rate of 5.6%. In a meta-analysis, it was concluded that, in general, a large group of vaginal surgery with and without mesh is associated with a higher risk of prolapse recurrence upon examination (RR 1.9 95% CI 1.3–2.7), of reoperation for prolapse recurrence (RR 2.3 95% CI 1.2–4.3), postoperative stress urinary incontinence (RR 1.9 95% CI 1.2–2.9) and dyspareunia (RR 2.5 95% 1.2–5.5) compared with sacrocolpopexy [29]. However, sacrocolpopexy was associated with a higher rate of paralytic ileus or small bowel obstruction (2.7% vs. 0.2%, $p < 0.01$), of complications related to intraperitoneal mesh or suture (4.2% vs. 0.4%, $p < 0.01$) and thromboembolic disease (0.6% vs. 0.1%, $p = .03$) [30].

The robotic sacrocolpopexy is the currently latest version of this technique. The robotic approach is associated with objective cure rates of 84% -100%, subjective cure rates of 92–95%, and a mesh erosion rate of 2% (range 0–8%). In general, we can find postoperative complications in this meta-analysis in up to 11% (range 0–43%), with serious complications in 2%, with a conversion rate of <1% to open surgery (range 0–5%) [31].

Traditionally, researchers have defined surgical success using anatomical results (POP-Q stage 0–1 - **Table 1**) and defined surgical failure as POPQ stage 2 or greater. More recently it is suggested that these anatomical definitions are too strict as more

Pelvic organ prolapse quantification system (POP-Q)	
Stage	**Description**
0	No prolapse, anterior and posterior points are all −3 cm, and C or D is between -TVL and -(TVL-2) cm
1	The criteria for stage 0 are not met, and the most distal prolapse is more than 1 cm above the level of the hymen (less than −1 cm)
2	The most distal prolapse if between 1 cm above and 1 cm below the hymen (at least one point is −1. 0, or + 1)
3	The most distal prolapse is more than 1 cm below the hymen but no further than 2 cm less than TVL
4	Represents complete procidentia or vault eversion; the most distal prolapse protrudes to at least (TVL-2) cm

Table 1.
POP-Q staging criteria.

than 75% of women presenting for annual gynecological exams with no symptoms of pelvic organ prolapse would not be found in the definition of "optimal anatomical result" and almost 40% would not meet the definition of "satisfactory anatomical result" [32]. The absence of symptoms of vaginal protrusion postoperatively has a significant relationship with the patient's evaluation of general improvement and improvement in quality of life after surgery, while anatomical success alone does not, and thus vaginal protrusion symptoms are of great importance when evaluating the surgical outcome of POP [11]. Another possible factor to take into account in the different studies is the concept of success used together with the POP classification used. Some authors have used the Baden-Walker prolapse classification system instead of the POP-Q, other studies have used a combination of anatomical criteria and the presence or absence of symptoms to define the success of the treatment. Such variability makes it difficult to compare the results between the different studies.

3. Case study

3.1 Aim and scope

In this study we will show the results obtained at our center with one of the most recent devices for the transvaginal correction of female POP, the Restorelle® single-incision mesh (Coloplast, USA). This product was later withdrawn from the market along with other transvaginal prosthetic devices for the correction of POP (April 2019), following its ban by the FDA.

Restorelle® Direct Fix Mesh products incorporate Smartmesh® technology (physiologically compatible ultralight mesh). It provides long-term strength while maintaining the vaginal elasticity of natural tissue. Its placement allows for an anterior sacrospinous ligament approach, using a disposable device (Digitex®) designed to place sutures without direct visualization. The proximal arms of the mesh are sutured to the anterior sacrospinous ligament and the distal arms of the mesh are sutured to the arch of the pelvic tendinous fascia.

3.2 Study design and material and methods

Retrospective study of patients who underwent surgical correction of POP in the same center between January 2016 and December 2017 with the Restorelle®

device. We analyzed demographic variables, prolapse characteristics, associated symptoms, gynecological history, recurrence, and degree of satisfaction taken from the existing medical history. The degree of POP was evaluated according to the Baden-Walker classification. The surgical indication was symptomatic patients with grade ≥ 2 POP (primary or recurrent). All interventions were performed by a single surgeon after an antibiotic prophylaxis protocol.

3.3 Results of the study

We retrospectively analyzed 78 patients operated on at our center with a mean age of 64.2 years (48–78). The comorbidities evaluated were diabetes mellitus (DM) (21%), arterial hypertension (48%), with a body mass index (BMI) of 27.5 kg/m^2 and a mean parity of 2.2 births (1–5). 36% of our patients had a history of gynecological surgical, the most prevalent being hysterectomy in up to 50% of the operated patients. The most frequently treated prolapse was anterior (72%), followed by posterior (12%) and mixed anterior–posterior (12%), with only one case of apical and posterior prolapse. Of these, 4 were recurrent prolapses. The most common grade of prolapse was III and IV with a frequency of 54% and 42%, respectively (**Table 2**).

Regarding the functional and clinical results, 50% of the sexually active patients had preoperative dyspareunia, which persisted after the intervention in two

Demographics	Variable value (n = 78)
Age (years)	64.2 (48–78)
BMI (kg/m2)	27.5 (21.9–33.3)
<25	13 (16.7%)
25–29.9	46 (59%)
>30 27	19 (24.4%)
DM	17 (21.8%)
Arterial hypertension	38 (48.7%)
Clinical history	
Parity	2.2 (1–5)
Previus gynecological operation	28 (36%)
Previous hysterectomy	14 (18%)
Previous POP surgery	4 (5.1%)
Pelvic organ prolapse	
Cystocele	57 (73.1%)
Rectocele	9 (11.5%)
Apex	1 (1.3%)
Mixed	11 (14.1%)
Grade	
Stage 2	2 (2.6%)
Stage 3	43 (55.1%)
Stage 4	33 (42.3%)

Values are presented as median [range] or number (%); BMI: body mass index; POP: pelvic organ prolapse.

Table 2.
Demographic variables and clinical characteristics before surgery.

Results	Preoperative	Postoperative
Dyspareunia	21 (26.9%)	2 (2.6%)
Urinary incontinence:	38 (48%)	24 (30.7%)
Urgency	29 (37.2%)	27 (34.6%)
Stress	24 (30.8%)	12 (15.4%)
Mixed	15 (19.2%)	8 (10.3%)
Unmasked UI		9 (11.5%)
Complications		
Extrusion	5 (6,4%)	
Pain	3 (3,8%)	
Functional recurrence	3 (3,8%)	
Anatomical recurrence	7 (9%)	

Table 3.
Results and complications during follow-up.

patients. Preoperative UI (urinary incontinence) was present in 48%, with urgency, stress UI and mixed UI in 37%, 31% and 19% respectively. 18% of these patients resolved their UI and 12% had postoperative UI (**Table 3**). We obtained a success rate of 92%, understood as absence of extrusion (6%), pain (3%) or functional recurrence (3%) 6 months after surgery. The anatomic recurrence rate was 9%. The total Clavien-Dindo IIIa complication rate was the most prevalent with 6.4% (extrusion), followed by grade II (3.8%). There were none in group IV or V. Cases of extrusion were resolved on an outpatient basis with local anesthesia. The mean follow-up time was 13.5 months. In general, the patients were satisfied (57.7%) or very satisfied (36%), and only 6.4% of the patients were dissatisfied and none were very dissatisfied.

4. Discussion

Surgical techniques can be performed using an abdominal or vaginal approach, depending on the medical history, physical examination, and experience of the surgeon. Laparoscopic sacrocolpopexy is an adequate therapeutic option with a high success rate in 80–100% of cases [33, 34]. However, this technique is not always appropriate, especially for patients who are at high risk for anesthesia, a multi-operated abdomen, or in recurrent prolapse. In these cases, a vaginal approach offers an interesting surgical alternative. Transvaginal mesh was developed to maintain the advantage of a vaginal procedure, while reducing the risk of recurrent prolapse compared to native tissue repair.

In the short and medium term, our results are similar to the articles published in relation to the success rate of studies with the same device and implantation route (92% in our series vs. 80.3%) [22] and different prosthetic devices but with the same implantation route (91.3%) [35], although its comparison is difficult due to the existence of different follow-up times. In our series, the minimum follow-up time was 6 months, while in studies such as the one published by Ferry et al. [22] they only had 3 months of follow-up. We could say that our success rate is slightly higher, despite a longer follow-up. Our good results may be due to the fact that all surgeries were performed by a single surgeon with extensive experience in vaginal

POP correction surgery with mesh interposition. If we compare other techniques with a recent boom, such as laparoscopic or robotic sacrocolpopexy [27, 28], there are also no great differences with respect to the success rate, 92% in our series versus 80–100% in those mentioned.

Our anatomical correction rate at 6 months of follow-up was 91%, similar to that found in other studies with this same device, 87.9% [22] or other light weight devices with the same implantation route, which oscillates between 79 and 96.5% [35–37], although their comparison is equally difficult due to different follow-up times. This same mesh surgery with the same anatomical correction rate criterion was 98.7% at 36 months for De Tayrac et al. [21] and 93.7% for Denance´ et al. [38]. Most of the published studies are retrospective [39], and those that are prospective have a follow-up period that is too short. If we compare other techniques such as robotic sacrocolpopexy [27], we find similar rates of absence of anatomic recurrence (95%).

Regarding the complications observed, the mesh extrusion rate in our series was 6.4% compared to 1.3–11.5% published in other studies with lightweight vaginal mesh (28 g / m2) [19, 21]. In a study published with the Restorelle® device, an extrusion rate of 2.8% was observed, lower than that obtained at our center. Again, this difference can be justified because the postsurgical follow-up at our center was more than double that of the referenced study [22]. Furthermore, in general, we can affirm that it is difficult to compare our data with the literature, as there is great diversity of previously available prosthetic products.

The functional results obtained are similar to those published to date. We can find postoperative dyspareunia in 1.76% of patients in some existing studies after the use of transvaginal mesh [36, 40], a rate very similar to that of our study with only two existing cases. In the case of laparoscopic sacrocolpopexy, there seems to be a lower risk of dyspareunia compared to the transvaginal implantation device (RR 0.39, 95% CI 0.18) [41, 42]. Incontinence rates were lower after correction of the prolapse, mainly, stress urinary incontinence improved [40, 43] and 12% of new cases appeared. On the other hand, the appearance of de novo stress urinary incontinence is common in the treatment of prolapse with the use of prosthetic material (RR 1.55, 95% CI 1.02 to 2.35 - anterior colporrhaphy versus use of transvaginal mesh), a fact that patients undergoing this surgery should always be advised of. However, our rate of de novo urinary incontinence with the use of transvaginal mesh is similar to that published with the laparoscopic colposacropexy technique (12%) [41].

Summarizing, we can state that transvaginal single incision-mesh have several advantages compared to classical approaches like colposacropexy or other mesh devices. It avoids the peritoneal cavity, truly important in patients with previous abdominal surgeries, reducing the risk of paralytic ileus and making possible a shorten recovery. As we have shown in our cases study, it can be done under locoregional anesthesia, allowing to perform this surgery almost without hospital stay. And finally, the esthetic results are obviously better, as we can avoid any abdominal scar, a fact that is especially transcendent in young women.

Our study presents several limitations. The first of these is the retrospective and non-randomized nature of our study. Furthermore, all the interventions were carried out by the same surgeon with great experience, which makes it difficult to reproduce these results in other centers and makes it difficult to compare them with other studies. On the other hand, the results of the treatments of non-oncological pathologies usually respond to very high expectations on behalf of the patients, so we can consider a limitation of our study the absence of quality of life questionnaires that assess the impact of success obtained after surgery and possible complications during follow-up.

5. Conclusion

In our experience, the Restorelle® device and its transvaginal placement is a safe procedure, with low morbidity and a high satisfaction rate in properly selected patients and in the hands of expert surgeons. Complications are rare and can be resolved by outpatient surgery.

Considering long-term complications is essential to properly weigh the risk–benefit ratio of each procedure, which is why more studies with a longer follow-up period than those currently available in the literature are necessary to judge this type of device with more evidence.

Conflict of interest

The authors declare no conflict of interest.

Appendices and nomenclature

BMI	Body mass index
DM	Diabetes mellitus
FDA	Food and Drug Administration
ICS	International Continence Society
IUGA	International Urogynecological Association
POP	pelvic organ prolapses
UI	urinary incontinence

Author details

Cristina Margarita Fernández-Ávila[1], Rodrigo García-Baquero[2*], Ana Victoria Ojeda Claro[3], Blanca Madurga Patuel[3] and José Luis Álvarez-Ossorio[4]

1 Urology Department, Hospital de La Línea de la Concepción, La Línea de la Concepción, Spain

2 Andrology and Reconstructive Urogenital Surgery Unit, Urology Department, Hospital Universitario Puerta del Mar, Cádiz, Spain

3 Functional Urology Unit, Urology Department, Hospital Universitario Puerta del Mar, Cádiz, Spain

4 Urology Department, Hospital Universitario Puerta del Mar, Cádiz, Spain

*Address all correspondence to: rgbaquero@hotmail.com

References

[1] Phillips CH, Anthony F, Benyon C, AK. M. Collagen metabolism in the uterosacral ligaments and vaginal skin in women with uterine prolapse. BJOG. 2006;113:39-46.

[2] Hodgkinson CP. Metallic bead-chain urethrocystography in preoperative and postoperative evaluation ofgynecologic urologic problems. Clin Obstet Gynecol. 1978; 21: 725-730.

[3] Barski D, Otto T, Gerullis H. Systematic review and classification of complications after anterior, posterior, apical, and total vaginal mesh implantation for prolapse repair. Surg Technol Int. 2014;24:217.

[4] European Commission, Directorate General for Health & Consumers. Opinion on the safety of surgical meshes used in urogynecological surgery. [Internet]. Luxembourg: European Commission; 2015 [citado 12 de octubre de 2019]. Disponible en: http://bookshop.europa.eu/uri?target=EUB:NOTICE:NDAS14005:EN:HTML

[5] Norton, P.A., Pelvic floor disorders: the role of fascia and ligaments. Clin Obstet Gynecol. 1993; 36(4): 926-938.

[6] DeLancey, J.O., The anatomy of the pelvic floor. Curr Opin Obstet Gynecol. 1994; 6(4): 313-316.

[7] Handa VL GE, Hendrix S, et al. Progression and remission of pelvic organ prolapse: a longitudinal study of menopausal women. Am J Obstet Gynecol. 2004;190(1):27-32.

[8] Aigmueller T DA, Hinterholzer S, Geiss I, Riss P. An estimation of the frequency of surgery for posthysterectomy vault prolapsed. Int Urogynecol J. 2010;21:299-302.

[9] Brown, J.S., et al., Pelvic organ prolapse surgery in the United States, 1997 Am J Obstet Gynecol. 2002; 186(4): 712-6.

[10] Ellerkmann RM, Cundiff GW, Melick CF, Nihira MA, Leffler K, Bent AE. Correlation of symptoms with location and severity of pelvic organ prolapse. American journal of obstetrics and gynecology. 2001;185(6):1332-7; discussion 1337- 8.

[11] Barber MD, Brubaker L, Nygaard I, Wheeler TL, 2nd, Schaffer J, Chen Z, et al. Defining success after surgery for pelvic organ prolapse. Obstetrics and gynecology. 2009;114(3):600-609.

[12] Madurga Patuel, M; et al. Documento de consenso de la asociación española de urología sobre la utilización de mallas en la cirugía del prolapso de órganos pélvicos [Internet] Spain: Asociación Española de Urología; 2019 [Citado Octubre 2019]. Available from: https://www.aeu.es/UserFiles/files/DocuAeuMallasCxPOP2019.pdf

[13] Olsen AL, Smith VJ, Bergstrom JO, Colling JC, Clark AL. Epidemiology of surgically managed pelvic organ prolapse and urinary incontinence. Obstetrics and gynecology. 1997;89(4):501-506.

[14] Weber AM, Walters MD, Piedmonte MR, Ballard LA. Anterior colporrhaphy: a randomized trial of three surgical techniques. American journal of obstetrics and gynecology. 2001;185(6):1299-1304.

[15] Denman M GW, Boyles S, Smith V, Edwards R, Clark A. 2008;198:555. Reoperation rate 10 years after surgically managed pelvic organ prolapse and urinary incontinence. American journal of obstetrics and gynecology. 2008;198:555.

[16] Sand PK, Koduri S, Lobel RW, Winkler HA, Tomezsko J, Culligan PJ,

et al. Prospective randomized trial of polyglactin 910 mesh to prevent recurrence of cystoceles and rectoceles. American journal of obstetrics and gynecology. 2001;184(7):1357-1362.

[17] Chmielewski L, Walters MD, Weber AM, Barber MD. Reanalysis of a randomized trial of 3 techniques of anterior colporrhaphy using clinically relevant definitions of success. American journal of obstetrics and gynecology. 2011.

[18] Julian TM. The efficacy of Marlex mesh in the repair of severe, recurrent vaginal prolapse of the anterior midvaginal wall. American journal of obstetrics and gynecology. 1996;175(6):1472-1475.

[19] Maher C, Feiner B, Baessler K, Christmann-Schmid C, Haya N, Marjoribanks J. Transvaginal mesh or grafts compared with native tissue repair for vaginal prolapse. The Cochrane database of systematic reviews. 2016;2:CD012079.

[20] Altman D, Mikkola TS, Bek KM, Rahkola-Soisalo P, Gunnarsson J, Engh ME, et al. Pelvic organ prolapse repair using the Uphold Vaginal Support System: a 1-year multicenter study. International urogynecology journal. 2016.

[21] De Tayrac R, Brouziyne M, Priou G, Devoldere G, Marie G, Renaudie J. Transvaginal repair of stage III-IV cystocele using a lightweight mesh: safety and 36-month outcome. International urogynecology journal. 2015;26(8):1147-1154.

[22] Ferry P, Bertherat P, Gauthier A, Villet R, Del Piano F, Hamid D, Fernandez H, Broux PL, Salet-Lizée D, Vincens E, Ntshaykolo P, Debodinance P, Pocholle P, Thirouard Y, de Tayrac R. Transvaginal treatment of anterior and apical genital prolapses using an Ultra lightweight mesh: Restorelle® Direct Fix™. A retrospective study on feasibility and morbidity. J Gynecol Obstet Hum Reprod. 2018 Nov;47(9):443-449.

[23] FDA. Urogynecologic Surgical Mesh: Update on the Safety and Effectiveness of Transvaginal Placement for Pelvic Organ Prolapse 2011 15/10/2013; (July 13,2011):[1-15 pp.]. Available from: http://www.fda.gov/downloads/MedicalDevices/Safety/AlertsandNotices/UCM262760.pdf.

[24] Gandhi S, Goldberg RP, Kwon C, Koduri S, Beaumont JL, Abramov Y, et al. A prospective randomized trial using solvent dehydrated fascia lata for the prevention of recurrent anterior vaginal wall prolapse. American journal of obstetrics and gynecology. 2005;192(5):1649-1654.

[25] Diwadkar GB, Barber MD, Feiner B, Maher C, Jelovsek JE. Complication and reoperation rates after apical vaginal prolapse surgical repair: a systematic review. Obstetrics and gynecology. 2009;113(2 Pt 1):367-373.

[26] Ow LL, Lim YN, Dwyer PL, Karmakar D, Murray C, Thomas E, et al. Native tissue repair or transvaginal mesh for recurrent vaginal prolapse: what are the long-term outcomes? International urogynecology journal. 2016.

[27] Higgs PJ, Chua HL, Smith AR, editors. Long term review of laparoscopic sacrocolpopexy. England 2005.

[28] Rivoire C, Botchorishvili R, Canis M, Jardon K, Rabischong B, Wattiez A, et al., editors. Complete laparoscopic treatment of genital prolapse with meshes including vaginal promontofixation and anterior repair: a series of 138 patients. United States 2007

[29] Maher C, Feiner B, Baessler K, Christmann-Schmid C, Haya N,

Brown J. Surgery for women with apical vaginal prolapse. Cochrane Database of Systematic Reviews. 2016(10).

[30] Siddiqui NY, Grimes CL, Casiano ER, Abed HT, Jeppson PC, Olivera CK, et al. Mesh sacrocolpopexy compared with native tissue vaginal repair: a systematic review and meta-analysis. Obstetrics and gynecology. 2015;125(1):44-55.

[31] Serati M, Bogani G, Sorice P, Braga A, Torella M, Salvatore S, et al. Robot-assisted sacrocolpopexy for pelvic organ prolapse: a systematic review and meta-analysis of comparative studies. European urology. 2014;66(2):303-318.

[32] Swift S, Woodman P, O'Boyle A, Kahn M, Valley M, Bland D, et al. Pelvic Organ Support Study (POSST): the distribution, clinical definition, and epidemiologic condition of pelvic organ support defects. American journal of obstetrics and gynecology. 2005;192(3):795-806.

[33] Lucot J-P, Fritel X, Debodinance P, Bader G, Cosson M, Giraudet G, et al. E'tude randomise'e comparant la promontofixation coelioscopique a` la chirurgie prothe´ tique par voie vaginale pour le traitement des cystoce` les: PROSPERE (PROSthetic PElvic organ prolapse REpair). J Gyne´ cologie Obste´ trique Biol Reprod. 2013;42(4):334-341.

[34] Park Y-H, Yang SC, Park ST, Park SH, Kim HB. Laparoscopic reconstructive surgery is superior to vaginal reconstruction in the pelvic organ prolapse. Int J Med Sci. 2014;11(11):1082-1088.

[35] Laso-García IM, Rodríguez-Cabello MA, Jiménez-Cidre MA, Orosa-Andrada A, Carracedo-Calvo D, López-Fando L, Burgos-Revilla FJ. Prospective long-term results, complications and risk factors in pelvic organ prolapse treatment with vaginal mesh. Eur J Obstet Gynecol Reprod Biol. 2017 Apr;211:62-67.

[36] Hinoul P, Ombelet WU, Burger MP, Roovers J-P. A prospective study to evaluate the anatomic and functional outcome of a transobturator mesh kit (prolift anterior) for symptomatic cystocele repair. J Minim Invasive Gynecol 2008;15 (January (5)):615-20.

[37] Khan ZA, Thomas L, Emery SJ. Outcomes and complications of trans-vaginal mesh repair using the ProliftTM kit for pelvic organ prolapse at 4 years median follow-up in a tertiary referral centre. Arch Gynecol Obstet 2014;290 (December (6)):1151-7.

[38] Denance´ M, Quiboeuf E, Hocke´ C. Results, safety and patient satisfaction at 6 months of vaginal anterior wall prolapse surgery by transvaginal repair with mesh use. Progres En Urol J Assoc Francaise Urol Soc Francaise Urol 2016;26(10):582-588.

[39] Unger CA, Barber MD. Vaginal mesh in pelvic reconstructive surgery: controversies, current use, and complications. Clin Obstet Gynecol 2015;58 (December (4)):740-53.

[40] Duport C, Duperron C, Delorme E. Anterior and middle pelvic organ prolapse repair using a six tension-free strap low weight transvaginal mesh: long-term retrospective monocentric study of 311 patients. J Gynecol Obstet Hum Reprod. 2019 Mar;48(3):143-149.

[41] Wei D, Wang P, Niu X, Zhao X. Comparison between laparoscopic uterus/sacrocolpopexy and total pelvic floor reconstruction with vaginal mesh for the treatment of pelvic organ prolapse. J Obstet Gynaecol Res. 2019 Apr;45(4):915-922.

[42] Coolen AWM, van IJsselmuiden MN, van Oudheusden AMJ, Veen J, van Eijndhoven HWF, Mol BWJ, Roovers JP,

Bongers MY. Laparoscopic sacrocolpopexy versus vaginal sacrospinous fixation for vaginal vault prolapse, a randomized controlled trial: SALTO-2 trial, study protocol. BMC Womens Health. 2017 Jul; 26;17(1):52.

[43] Van Raalte HM, Lucente VR, Molden SM, Haff R, Murphy M. One-year anatomic and quality-of-life outcomes after the Prolift procedure for treatment of posthysterectomy prolapse. Am J Obstet Gynecol. 2008;199(December (6)) 694. e1-694. e6.